# THE AI HEALTHCARE REVOLUTION

**T.C. Catz**
**The AI Healthcare Revolution**



Published by Spines
ISBN: 979-8-89569-734-4

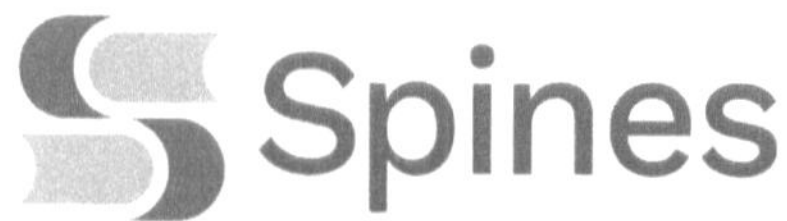

# The AI Healthcare Revolution

## Integrating Technology for Enhanced Patient Solutions

T.C. Catz

# Contents

# Dedication

*This book is dedicated to all those who have dedicated their lives to improving healthcare, to the pioneers of artificial intelligence who paved the way for this revolutionary transformation, and to the patients who inspire us with their resilience and courage. May this work serve as a testament to their tireless efforts and a beacon of hope for a healthier future.*

# PREFACE

The field of healthcare is on the cusp of a profound revolution, driven by the transformative power of artificial intelligence (AI). This book embarks on a journey into the exciting landscape where AI is reshaping medical practices, empowering doctors with unparalleled tools, and offering patients a brighter future.

As we delve into the intricacies of AI's impact on healthcare, we will explore its diverse applications, from revolutionizing diagnosis and treatment to personalizing patient care and enhancing the overall patient experience. We will examine the ethical considerations that accompany this technological advancement, ensuring responsible and equitable integration of AI in healthcare.

This book is designed to be accessible to a wide audience, from healthcare professionals seeking to integrate AI into their practices to patients curious about its potential benefits and those simply interested in the future of medicine. With a multi-faceted approach, we aim to provide a comprehensive overview of AI's role in healthcare, its transformative potential, and the exciting possibilities it holds for a healthier tomorrow.

# INTRODUCTION

Imagine a world where diseases are diagnosed with unprecedented accuracy, treatment plans are tailored to individual needs, and healthcare is readily accessible to everyone. This is the future that artificial intelligence (AI) promises to bring to the world of healthcare.

AI is no longer a futuristic concept, but a powerful force rapidly transforming the medical landscape. From analyzing complex medical images to identifying subtle patterns in patient data, AI is empowering healthcare professionals with new tools to diagnose diseases earlier, personalize treatment, and improve patient outcomes.

This book serves as your guide to the exciting and transformative world of AI in healthcare. We will explore the fundamental concepts of AI, delve into its diverse applications in medical diagnosis, treatment, and patient care, and discuss the ethical considerations that accompany this revolutionary technology. We will journey through the exciting possibilities of AI in the operating room, the power of data in transforming patient care, and the role of AI in enhancing the patient experience.

This book is not merely about technology, but about people. It is about how AI can empower healthcare professionals to provide better care, how it can empower patients to take control of their health, and how it can ultimately shape a healthier future for everyone.

# Why The N.E.R.D.Y. Way?

The **N.E.R.D.Y.** Way, a potent acronym that stands for kNowledge, Education, Resource, Discovery for You, embodies the spirit of this book. It's not just a journey through the world of AI; it's an invitation to embark on a lifelong adventure of learning, exploration, and constant evolution. As the field of AI progresses at an astonishing pace, so too must our understanding and engagement with it. The NERDY Way encourages you to embrace this dynamic and ever-changing landscape as a catalyst for personal growth and societal advancement.

Think of it as an ongoing dialogue, a conversation between you and the world of AI, where curiosity is your compass and exploration is your guide. This journey is not about reaching a destination; it's about the continuous process of learning, adapting, and evolving alongside the ever-expanding frontiers of AI. Embrace the challenges and opportunities that come with this journey, for within them lies the potential to unlock your own capabilities and contribute to a future where technology empowers humanity.

The N.E.R.D.Y. Way is a mindset, a philosophy that encourages you to approach AI with a sense of wonder and a spirit of inquiry. It's about recognizing the profound impact AI is having on every aspect of our lives and acknowledging its potential to reshape our world. This mindset fosters a deep appreciation for the transformative power of AI while also recognizing the critical need for responsible development and deployment. It's about understanding the intricate workings of AI systems, their strengths, and limitations, and using this knowledge to make informed decisions about their use.

The N.E.R.D.Y. Way isn't just about acquiring knowledge; it's about applying it to create a better future. This journey is about using your understanding of AI to solve global challenges, foster collaboration between humans and machines, and shape a future where technology serves as a force for good. It's about embracing the responsibility that comes with this knowledge, recognizing that AI's future depends on our collective efforts.

For those who choose to embark on this journey, the rewards are boundless. You will gain a deeper understanding of the world around you, develop valuable skills, and contribute to a future where technology serves as a force for good. It's an invitation to join the conversation, to contribute to the dialogue, and to shape the future of AI for the benefit of all. The N.E.R.D.Y. Way is a testament to the power of learning, collaboration, and continuous exploration, a journey that will enrich your life and help build a better future for everyone.

The N.E.R.D.Y. Way isn't just about understanding AI; it's about becoming a part of its evolution, a contributor to its progress, and a champion for its responsible development and deployment. It's a reminder that the future of AI is not a distant prospect; it's happening now, and it's up to us to shape it. It's a call to action, a reminder that we all have a role to play in this journey, and every step we take, every question we ask, every idea we share, helps us move closer to a brighter future.

CHAPTER 1

---

# THE DAWN OF AI IN HEALTHCARE

## A WORLD TRANSFORMED

The dawn of artificial intelligence (AI) has cast a long shadow over the landscape of healthcare, ushering in an era of transformative change. This burgeoning technology holds immense potential to revolutionize medical practices, empowering doctors with unprecedented tools to diagnose diseases with remarkable accuracy, predict potential complications, and personalize treatment plans like never before.

AI's journey began in the mid-20th century, with the birth of the first computer programs designed to mimic human intelligence. These early forays into AI were largely theoretical, fueled by the visionary ideas of mathematicians and computer scientists who sought to unlock the secrets of the human mind. In the 1960s and 1970s, the field witnessed a surge of interest in AI applications, particularly in the field of medicine. Researchers explored the use of AI for medical diagnosis, with the development of expert systems capable of analyzing patient symptoms and suggesting potential diagnoses.

The early applications of AI in medicine were often limited by the constraints of computing power and data availability. However, these pioneering efforts laid the foundation for the remarkable advancements that would come to shape the future of healthcare. The emergence of big data in the early 21st century marked a pivotal turning point, providing AI with the fuel it needed to truly take off. With the vast accumulation of medical data from electronic health records, medical imaging scans, and wearable devices, AI algorithm gained the ability to learn from patterns and make predictions with unprecedented accuracy.

The early 2000s saw the rise of machine learning, a subfield of AI that focuses on enabling computers to learn from data without explicit programming. Machine learning algorithms were able to analyze massive datasets, identifying hidden correlations and making predictions that could revolutionize medical diagnosis and treatment. The development of deep learning algorithms, a subset of machine learning inspired by the structure of the human brain, further propelled AI's capabilities. Deep learning algorithms were particularly well-suited for analyzing complex patterns in medical images, such as mammograms, retinal scans, and tissue biopsies. These algorithms were able to detect subtle abnormalities that might be missed by the human eye, leading to earlier diagnosis and improved treatment outcomes.

The transformative potential of AI in healthcare was quickly recognized by researchers and practitioners alike. AI-powered systems began to emerge across various medical specialties, including radiology, oncology, cardiology, and ophthalmology. In radiology, deep learning algorithms were used to detect breast cancer in mammograms, identifying tumors that were previously missed by radiologists. In ophthalmology, AI systems were deployed to detect diabetic retinopathy in retinal scans, a leading cause of blindness in adults. These early successes in medical imaging demonstrated the power of AI to enhance diagnostic accuracy and improve patient outcomes.

Beyond medical imaging, AI has found its way into other areas of healthcare, including patient management, drug discovery, and surgical procedures. AI-powered systems are being used to analyze patient data from electronic health records, identifying trends and patterns that can help predict future health risks. This data-driven approach enables healthcare providers to proactively manage patient health, preventing complications and reducing the need for hospitalization.

AI is also playing a critical role in drug discovery, accelerating the process of identifying new drug targets and developing novel therapies. By analyzing vast amounts of data on chemical compounds and their potential interactions with biological systems, AI algorithms can predict which compounds are most likely to be effective as drugs. This ability to speed up drug discovery has the potential to revolutionize the pharmaceutical industry and bring new treatments to patients faster than ever before.

In the realm of surgery, AI is transforming surgical procedures, enabling surgeons to perform complex operations with greater precision and control. AI-powered robotic systems are being used to assist surgeons in performing minimally invasive procedures, reducing the need for large incisions and leading to faster recovery times. Image-guided surgery, another AI-powered innovation, uses real-time imaging to guide surgical instruments, ensuring greater accuracy and minimizing the risk of complications.

The applications of AI in healthcare are rapidly expanding, opening up new possibilities for improving patient care and shaping the future of medicine. However, with these advancements come ethical considerations that must be carefully addressed. Concerns have been raised about data privacy, algorithmic bias, and the potential for AI to displace healthcare professionals.

It is essential to ensure that AI is developed and deployed responsibly, with a focus on patient safety, fairness transparency. By addressing these ethical challenges head-on, we can harness the transformative power of AI to create a healthier future for everyone.

The dawn of AI in healthcare marks a new chapter in the history of medicine. As this technology continues to evolve, we can expect to see even more remarkable advancements in the coming years. The future of healthcare is filled with both promise and challenges, and it is up to us to ensure that AI is used to its full potential to improve the lives of patients worldwide.

## The Power of Data

The power of data is the lifeblood of AI in healthcare, enabling machines to learn, predict, and ultimately transform how we approach medicine. Imagine a world where vast amounts of patient information, from medical records to genetic sequences, are meticulously analyzed to reveal hidden patterns and unlock previously unimaginable insights. This is the world of big data in healthcare, and it is revolutionizing every facet of medical practice.

But where does this data come from, and how is it harnessed to train AI models? The answer lies in a complex tapestry of sources and technologies.

## The Data Tapestry: Weaving a Path to Understanding

Electronic health records (EHRs) are the cornerstone of big data in healthcare. These digital repositories store a wealth of patient information, including medical history, diagnoses, medications, and lab results. The sheer volume of data accumulated in EHRs is staggering, providing a rich tapestry of information for AI algorithms to analyze.

Beyond EHRs, a multitude of other sources contribute to the data deluge. Wearable devices, such as smartwatches and fitness trackers, track our heart rate, sleep patterns, and physical activity, offering real-time insights into our health and behavior. Social media data can reveal valuable information about health trends, disease outbreaks, and patient experiences. Even environmental data, such as air pollution levels and weather patterns, can contribute to a comprehensive understanding of health outcomes.

## Unveiling the Secrets: Analyzing Big Data

The raw data itself is meaningless without the tools to analyze it. This is where powerful data analytics techniques come into play. Machine learning algorithms, specifically deep learning models, are trained on these massive datasets to identify complex patterns and relationships. These algorithms can sift through millions of data points, identifying subtle correlations and anomalies that might escape the human eye.

For example, a deep learning model might be trained on a dataset of mammograms to identify subtle variations in tissue density that could indicate the presence of breast cancer. The model learns to recognize these patterns by analyzing thousands of mammograms, both cancerous and benign. Once trained, the model can then analyze new mammograms, identifying potential tumors with remarkable accuracy.

## Training the Machine: The Power of Data

Training an AI model is a complex process that involves feeding the model with vast amounts of data. This data serves as the model's "training ground," allowing it to learn the patterns and relationships that define a particular medical condition. The more data the model is trained on, the more accurate and reliable it becomes.

For example, an AI model designed to predict the risk of diabetic retinopathy might be trained on a dataset of millions of retinal scans. The model would analyze these scans, learning to identify the specific features that correlate with the development of this eye disease. Once trained, the model could then be used to screen individuals for early signs of diabetic retinopathy, enabling timely intervention and preventing vision loss.

## The Ethical Landscape: Navigating the Data Revolution

The use of big data in healthcare is not without its challenges. Privacy concerns are paramount, as vast amounts of sensitive patient information are being collected and analyzed. Ensuring data security and protecting patient confidentiality is crucial. Algorithmic bias is another concern, as AI models trained on biased data can perpetuate inequalities and perpetuate existing healthcare disparities.

## Beyond the Data: Human Expertise Remains Vital

While big data and AI offer immense potential, it's important to remember that they are tools, not replacements for human expertise. Doctors, nurses, and other healthcare professionals play a crucial role in interpreting AI-generated results, making clinical decisions, and providing compassionate care. AI can augment human capabilities, but it cannot replace the human touch.

## The Future of Data in Healthcare

The future of AI in healthcare is inextricably linked to the continued growth and sophistication of big data. As technology advances, we can expect to see even more data sources integrated into the healthcare ecosystem. This will create even greater opportunities for AI to enhance diagnosis, personalize treatment, and improve patient outcomes.

## From EHRs to Wearables: A Data-Driven Revolution

The healthcare landscape is undergoing a profound transformation, driven by the power of data. From the vast repositories of electronic health records to the real-time insights offered by wearable devices, data is becoming an essential component of modern medicine.

## A Sea of Information: Navigating the Data Ocean

Imagine a vast ocean of data, constantly expanding with new information. This is the reality of big data in healthcare. Every patient encounter, every diagnostic test, every wearable device generates data, contributing to this ever-growing ocean of information.

## The Data Engine: Powering AI in Healthcare

The data engine, fueled by advanced algorithms, is at the heart of AI in healthcare. These algorithms can navigate this sea of information, identifying patterns, making predictions, and providing insights that can revolutionize patient care.

## The Data Revolution: Empowering Patients and Providers

The data revolution in healthcare is not just about accumulating information; it's about harnessing the power of data to improve patient outcomes, empower patients with personalized care, and enhance the efficiency of healthcare delivery.

## Data-Driven Decision Making: A New Era of Healthcare

The ability to analyze vast amounts of data allows for data-driven decision-making in healthcare, leading to more accurate diagnoses, more effective treatment plans, and more personalized care for patients.

## Big Data and AI: A Synergistic Partnership

Big data and AI are not independent forces; they are a powerful partnership. Big data provides the raw material, the fuel for AI algorithms, while AI provides the intelligence, the ability to analyze and extract meaningful insights from this data.

## The Future of Healthcare: Data-Driven and AI-Enabled

The future of healthcare is data-driven and AI-enabled. As technology advances and data sources grow, AI will play an increasingly vital role in transforming every aspect of medical practice, from disease prevention to personalized treatment.

**A Data-Driven Future: Shaping a Healthier World**

The power of data, combined with the intelligence of AI, holds the potential to create a healthier world. By harnessing the insights derived from vast amounts of patient information, we can improve healthcare delivery, prevent disease, and ultimately enhance the lives of millions of people.

## MACHINE LEARNING

Machine learning, a subset of artificial intelligence (AI), forms the bedrock of AI's transformative impact on healthcare. It empowers computers to learn from data, identify patterns, and make predictions without explicit programming. This ability to learn from vast amounts of medical data has unlocked unprecedented possibilities in diagnostics, treatment, and patient care.

At its core, machine learning relies on algorithms that analyze data and adjust their parameters to improve performance. These algorithms are trained on massive datasets, enabling them to recognize intricate patterns and make accurate predictions. Different types of machine learning algorithms cater to diverse applications in healthcare, each offering unique strengths and capabilities:

1. **Supervised Learning:** This approach involves training algorithms on labeled data, where each data point is associated with a known outcome. Supervised learning algorithms learn to map inputs to outputs, making them particularly well-suited for tasks such as:
   - **Predicting disease risk:** By analyzing a patient's medical history, genetic information, and lifestyle factors, supervised learning models can estimate

the likelihood of developing specific diseases. This information empowers healthcare professionals to proactively identify patients at higher risk and implement preventive measures.

- **Diagnosing diseases:** Supervised learning algorithms can analyze medical images, lab results, and patient data to identify patterns associated with specific diseases. This enables early detection, faster diagnosis, and more accurate treatment planning.
- **Predicting treatment response:** Supervised learning models can analyze patient characteristics and treatment history to predict how individuals will respond to specific medications or therapies. This personalized approach optimizes treatment strategies and improves outcomes.

2. **Unsupervised Learning:** In contrast to supervised learning, unsupervised learning algorithms operate on unlabeled data, uncovering hidden patterns and structures within the data without prior knowledge of the outcomes. This approach is particularly effective for tasks such as:
   - **Clustering patients:** Unsupervised learning algorithms can group patients based on their characteristics, medical history, and treatment responses, leading to a better understanding of disease subgroups and tailored treatment approaches.
   - **Identifying anomalies:** These algorithms can detect unusual patterns in medical data, potentially indicating early signs of disease or complications.

This capability is particularly valuable in early disease detection and risk assessment.

- **Discovering new drug targets:** By analyzing large datasets of genomic and proteomic data, unsupervised learning algorithms can identify novel targets for drug development, accelerating the process of discovering new therapies.

- **Reinforcement Learning:** This type of machine learning involves training algorithms to learn from trial and error, optimizing their actions based on rewards and penalties.Reinforcement learning algorithms are particularly valuable in:

  - **Robot-assisted surgery:** Algorithms learn from previous surgeries, optimizing robot movements, instrument control, and minimizing tissue damage. This approach holds immense potential for enhancing precision and safety in surgical procedures.

  - **Personalized treatment planning:** Algorithms can learn from patient responses to different treatment strategies, optimizing treatment plans based on individual needs and maximizing therapeutic outcomes.

  - **Drug discovery and development:** Reinforcement learning can optimize the design of new drugs and therapies by iteratively adjusting their structure and properties based on their effectiveness and safety profiles.

## The Power of Machine Learning in Action

The real-world applications of machine learning in healthcare are already making a tangible impact on patient care. Here are some compelling examples:

- **Early Detection of Cancer:** AI-powered algorithms are revolutionizing cancer diagnosis by identifying subtle abnormalities in medical images that might be missed by human eyes. In mammography, AI algorithms can detect early signs of breast cancer with significantly higher accuracy than traditional methods, potentially leading to earlier detection and improved treatment outcomes.

- **Diabetic Retinopathy Screening:** Diabetic retinopathy, a leading cause of blindness, can be effectively detected and managed with early intervention. AI-powered systems are capable of analyzing retinal scans to identify early signs of damage, enabling prompt treatment and preventing vision loss.

- **Personalized Medicine:** Machine learning is transforming the practice of medicine by enabling personalized treatment plans based on individual patient characteristics. By analyzing genomic data, medical history, and lifestyle factors, AI algorithms can predict how individuals will respond to specific medications and treatments, ensuring optimal therapy and maximizing therapeutic outcomes.

- **AI-Powered Robotics in Surgery:** The integration of AI into surgical robotics is leading to more precise, minimally invasive procedures. AI algorithms can analyze real-time data during surgery, guiding robotic instruments with unprecedented accuracy and control, minimizing tissue damage and reducing recovery time.

- **Predictive Analytics for Patient Care:** Machine learning algorithms are being used to analyze electronic health records and identify patients at risk for developing specific diseases or complications. This enables healthcare professionals to proactively intervene and implement preventive measures, improving patient outcomes and reducing healthcare costs.

## The Ethical Implications of AI in Healthcare

While the potential benefits of machine learning in healthcare are immense, it is crucial to acknowledge and address the ethical implications of its application. Key concerns include:

- **Data Privacy and Security:** The use of AI in healthcare relies on the collection and analysis of sensitive patient data, raising concerns about privacy and security. Robust safeguards must be in place to protect patient information from unauthorized access and misuse.

- **Algorithmic Bias:** Machine learning algorithms are trained on data that reflects existing societal biases, potentially perpetuating inequalities in healthcare. It is essential to develop and implement methods to identify and mitigate algorithmic bias, ensuring fair and equitable access to healthcare for all.

- **Transparency and Explainability:** The complex nature of machine learning algorithms can make it difficult to understand how they arrive at their decisions. This lack of transparency can raise concerns about accountability and trust. Efforts are underway to develop more transparent and explainable AI models, enhancing trust and ensuring responsible use.

- **Job Displacement:** The automation of tasks through AI could potentially lead to job displacement in healthcare. It is crucial to proactively address this challenge by developing training programs for healthcare professionals to adapt to the evolving landscape of AI-driven healthcare.

## Conclusion

Machine learning is a transformative force in healthcare, empowering doctors with powerful tools for diagnosis, treatment, and patient care. By analyzing vast amounts of medical data, machine learning algorithms are revolutionizing diagnostic accuracy, personalizing treatment plans, and improving patient outcomes. However, it is essential to proceed with caution and address the ethical implications of this technology, ensuring responsible development and deployment for the benefit of all. As AI continues to advance, the future of healthcare holds immense promise for a more personalized, precise, and efficient system that prioritizes patient well-being. continues to advance, the future of healthcare holds immense promise for a more personalized, precise, and efficient system that prioritizes patient well-being.

## Deep Learning

Deep learning, a subfield of machine learning, emerges as a powerful tool in healthcare, capable of unlocking the complexities of medical data. While machine learning algorithms can identify patterns in relatively simple datasets, deep learning excels in handling intricate and high-dimensional information, enabling it to decipher the nuances of medical images and decipher the intricacies of human language.

At the heart of deep learning are artificial neural networks, inspired by the structure and function of the human brain.

These networks consist of interconnected layers of nodes, each processing and transmitting information. The architecture of these networks, akin to the intricate pathways of the brain, allows for the extraction of complex features from data. Through a process called "training," the network learns to identify patterns and relationships within the data, becoming adept at recognizing subtle abnormalities or predicting potential outcomes.

### Image Analysis: Unveiling the Hidden World of Medical Scans

Deep learning shines brightly in the field of medical imaging, transforming the way we analyze scans and diagnose diseases. Radiologists, tasked with interpreting intricate images, often rely on years of experience to identify subtle anomalies. Deep learning algorithms, trained on vast datasets of medical images, can detect these subtle patterns that may escape the human eye.

Consider the realm of mammography, where early detection of breast cancer is crucial for successful treatment.

Traditional mammograms, read by human radiologists, often miss small tumors, particularly in dense breast tissue. Deep learning algorithms, trained on thousands of mammograms, have shown remarkable ability to identify cancerous lesions with higher accuracy than human experts, potentially leading to earlier diagnoses and improved survival rates.

Beyond mammograms, deep learning's impact extends to other imaging modalities. Retinal scans, crucial for identifying diabetic retinopathy, benefit significantly from deep learning algorithms. These algorithms, trained on images of healthy and diseased retinas, can detect subtle changes in blood vessels and other structures that may indicate early stages of the disease, enabling timely intervention and preserving vision.

## Natural Language Processing: Bridging the Gap Between Human and Machine

Deep learning is not limited to image analysis; it's also revolutionizing the way we interact with medical data and information. Natural language processing (NLP), a field within AI that focuses on enabling computers to understand and interpret human language, leverages deep learning to unlock the vast potential of text-based medical data.

Electronic health records (EHRs), repositories of detailed patient information, contain a wealth of valuable data, but their sheer volume and complex structure make it challenging for humans to analyze efficiently. Deep learning algorithms can effectively process this textual data, extracting vital insights that can improve patient care.

One promising application lies in automated diagnosis. Deep learning algorithms can analyze patient records, identifying patterns associated with specific conditions, potentially assisting doctors in making accurate diagnoses. Furthermore, these algorithms can process medical literature and research papers, providing valuable insights and recommendations for treatment strategies.

## The Rise of Personalized Medicine

Beyond diagnosis, deep learning is paving the way for personalized medicine, tailoring treatment plans to individual patient needs. By analyzing patient data, including genetic information, medical history, and lifestyle factors, deep-learning algorithms can predict an individual's response to specific drugs or therapies.

Imagine a future where patients receive personalized treatment plans based on their unique genetic makeup and risk profiles, ensuring that they receive the most effective and safe treatment options. Deep learning is playing a crucial role in bringing this future to life, enabling physicians to make more informed decisions about patient care.

## Navigating the Challenges

While the potential of deep learning in healthcare is immense, there are challenges to address. The need for large datasets and robust computational power remains a concern.

Additionally, ethical considerations, such as privacy concerns, algorithmic bias, and the need for transparency, require careful attention. Moreover, deep learning models are often "black boxes," meaning that their decision-making processes can be opaque, making it difficult to understand why they make certain predictions. This lack of transparency poses challenges for trust and accountability.

**The Future of Deep Learning in Healthcare**

Despite the challenges, the future of deep learning in healthcare appears bright. Researchers are continuously developing new algorithms and techniques, pushing the boundaries of what AI can achieve. The advent of quantum computing promises to further enhance the capabilities of deep learning, enabling the analysis of even more complex datasets and leading to breakthroughs in medical research.

The integration of deep learning into clinical practice is transforming the healthcare landscape, empowering doctors with powerful tools to diagnose diseases, predict outcomes, and personalize treatment plans. As deep learning continues to evolve, we can expect even more transformative applications, leading to a future of more accurate diagnoses, personalized therapies, and improved patient care.

## Ethical Considerations and Challenges

The dawn of AI in healthcare brings immense promise, but it also raises profound ethical questions that must be addressed with utmost care. As AI algorithms become increasingly sophisticated and integrated into medical practices, it is crucial to ensure their responsible development and deployment. We must navigate this technological revolution with a keen awareness of the potential risks and benefits.

One of the most pressing ethical concerns is **Privacy** - AI systems rely on vast amounts of patient data, including medical records, genetic information, and even personal habits. The potential for misuse or unauthorized access to this sensitive data poses a significant threat to patient confidentiality. Robust data security measures are essential to safeguard patient privacy and prevent breaches that could have devastating consequences.

Another crucial ethical consideration is **algorithmic bias** - AI algorithms are trained on massive datasets, and if these datasets contain biases, those biases can be amplified and reflected in the algorithms' decisions. For instance, if a diagnostic algorithm is trained on data that predominantly represents a certain demographic group, it may be less accurate in diagnosing diseases in individuals from other groups. This could lead to disparities in healthcare outcomes and exacerbate existing health inequities.

The development and deployment of AI in healthcare must be **transparent and accountable** - Clear guidelines and regulations are needed to ensure that AI algorithms are developed and deployed responsibly. Transparency is essential to build trust in AI systems and allow for public scrutiny of their decision-making processes. This transparency should extend to the data used to train algorithms, the algorithms themselves, and the decision-making processes based on their output.

**Accountability** is also crucial. It is essential to identify who is responsible for the decisions made by AI algorithms. In cases where an AI system makes a mistake, it is important to determine who is accountable for the consequences. This requires clear protocols for oversight, governance, and accountability to ensure that AI systems are used safely and effectively.

Moreover, the **responsible use of AI in healthcare** necessitates a thoughtful approach to patient engagement and informed consent. Patients should be informed about the use of AI in their care and given the opportunity to consent to the use of their data. This is particularly important when using AI for diagnosis or treatment decisions, as these decisions can have a significant impact on a patient's life.

The ethical considerations surrounding AI in healthcare are complex and multifaceted. There is no one-size-fits-all solution, and ongoing dialogue and collaboration are needed to address the challenges and ensure that AI is used ethically and responsibly. This includes collaboration between healthcare professionals, researchers, policymakers, and the public to develop robust frameworks and guidelines for the development and deployment of AI in healthcare.

It is crucial to recognize that **AI is a tool** – a powerful tool with the potential to revolutionize healthcare and improve patient outcomes. However, like any tool, AI must be used responsibly and ethically. We must strive to develop and implement AI systems that are fair, transparent, and accountable, ensuring that they benefit all patients and promote equity in healthcare.

The promise of AI in healthcare is undeniable. It has the potential to unlock new insights, improve diagnostics, personalize treatment plans, and ultimately transform the way we care for patients. However, we must approach this technological revolution with caution and a commitment to ethical principles. By addressing the ethical challenges and ensuring the responsible use of AI, we can harness its power to create a healthier future for all.

CHAPTER 2

---

# AI-POWERED DIAGNOSIS

## REVOLUTIONIZING DETECTION UNMASKING HIDDEN PATTERNS

## UNMASKING HIDDEN PATTERNS

Imagine peering into the intricate details of a medical scan, the kind that reveals the inner workings of our bodies. For years, radiologists have been the guardians of these images, their expert eyes trained to discern subtle abnormalities that could signal the presence of disease. But now, a new era is dawning, one where artificial intelligence (AI) joins the ranks of medical experts, bringing a revolutionary level of precision to the task of diagnosis.

AI, with its extraordinary ability to analyze vast amounts of data and detect patterns that might escape the human eye, is transforming the field of medical imaging. It's not about replacing human expertise, but rather augmenting it, empowering doctors with powerful tools to see beyond the limitations of their own vision.

Take the realm of mammography, where detecting breast cancer early can significantly improve a woman's chances of survival. AI algorithms are now being trained on massive datasets of mammograms, learning to identify subtle, telltale signs of malignancy that might have been missed by human eyes. These algorithms are capable of analyzing thousands of mammograms in mere minutes, flagging suspicious areas for further review by radiologists. This allows radiologists to focus their attention on the most critical cases, potentially leading to earlier detection and intervention.

The story of AI in medical imaging is not limited to breast cancer. Diabetic retinopathy, a leading cause of blindness in adults, can be effectively treated if detected early. AI-powered systems are now being used to analyze retinal scans, identifying subtle changes in blood vessels and other indicators of the disease. These systems can flag patients at risk for diabetic retinopathy, allowing for timely interventions and preventing potentially devastating vision loss.

But the power of AI extends beyond the realm of visible images. Pathologists, who analyze tissue samples to diagnose diseases, are also embracing the transformative potential of AI. Imagine a pathologist peering through a microscope, meticulously examining tissue samples for signs of cancer. This process can be time-consuming and prone to human error. Now, AI algorithms are being trained to analyze these tissue samples, identifying specific biomarkers and patterns that can help with diagnosis and prognosis.

AI can analyze vast numbers of slides, detecting subtle variations in cell morphology and other features that might elude the human eye. This allows pathologists to focus their expertise on the most complex cases, potentially leading to faster and more accurate diagnoses.

The applications of AI in medical imaging are vast and growing. Beyond mammograms and retinal scans, AI is being used to analyze images from CT scans, MRIs, and ultrasounds. It is helping doctors identify abnormalities in the brain, heart, lungs, and other organs, leading to earlier detection and improved treatment outcomes.

The impact of AI on medical imaging is profound. It's about empowering doctors with new tools, enhancing their diagnostic accuracy, and ultimately improving patient care. The future of medical imaging is bright, with AI playing an increasingly critical role in revolutionizing detection and shaping a healthier future for all.

## Early Detection

Imagine a world where diseases are detected before they even show symptoms, where treatments are tailored to each individual's unique needs, and where healthcare is accessible to everyone, regardless of location or socioeconomic status.

This is the future that AI is paving the way for, and early detection is at the heart of this revolution.

AI-powered systems are emerging as powerful tools for identifying subtle changes in medical data, allowing for earlier and more precise diagnosis. By analyzing large datasets of medical images, patient records, and even genetic information, AI algorithms can spot patterns that may be missed by the human eye. This ability to identify early signs of disease is transforming healthcare, offering the promise of improved treatment outcomes and potentially even preventing the onset of serious conditions.

One of the most prominent examples of AI's impact on early detection is in the field of breast cancer. AI algorithms are being used to analyze mammograms, identifying suspicious areas that may be missed by radiologists. Studies have shown that these AI-powered systems can increase the accuracy of breast cancer detection by up to 15%, leading to earlier diagnosis and potentially saving lives.

The benefits of AI-powered early detection extend beyond breast cancer. AI systems are proving effective in diagnosing other life-threatening conditions like diabetic retinopathy, a leading cause of blindness in adults. By analyzing retinal scans, AI algorithms can identify subtle changes in the blood vessels and other structures of the eye, providing an early warning sign of the disease. Early intervention through laser treatment or other therapies can significantly reduce the risk of vision loss.

The power of AI in early detection goes beyond medical imaging. AI systems are being used to analyze electronic health records, identifying patients at risk for heart disease, stroke, and other conditions based on their medical history, lifestyle factors, and genetic predispositions. This allows healthcare providers to take proactive steps to prevent these diseases, such as recommending lifestyle changes, screening tests, or preventative medications.

The development of AI-powered early detection systems is driven by the increasing availability of large datasets and advancements in machine learning algorithms. The ability of AI to analyze massive amounts of data and identify complex patterns is crucial to its success in detecting early signs of disease.

However, it's important to note that AI is not a replacement for human expertise. Doctors and other healthcare professionals remain essential in interpreting AI-generated results, making treatment decisions, and providing patient care. AI acts as a powerful tool to enhance human capabilities, not to replace them.

The use of AI in early detection is still evolving, and there are ongoing efforts to improve the accuracy and reliability of these systems. Researchers are working to address challenges such as algorithmic bias, ensuring that AI systems are not inadvertently discriminating against certain groups of patients.

Despite the challenges, the potential of AI in early detection is undeniable. As AI technology continues to advance, we can expect to see even more sophisticated systems capable of identifying diseases earlier and more accurately, leading to better treatment outcomes and improving the health and well-being of patients worldwide.

The story of AI in early detection is just beginning. It is a story of innovation, collaboration, and the relentless pursuit of improving human health. It is a story that is being written every day, as researchers and healthcare professionals work together to unlock the full potential of AI to make a real difference in the lives of patients. This is a story of hope, of a future where diseases are detected early, treated effectively, and prevented whenever possible.

## AI in Pathology

The realm of pathology, the study of diseases, has traditionally relied on meticulous manual analysis of tissue samples under microscopes. This process, while invaluable, is time-consuming, prone to human error, and often limited by the subjective interpretations of individual pathologists. However, a new era of precision is dawning, fueled by the power of artificial intelligence (AI).

AI is transforming the landscape of pathology, bringing with it the potential to revolutionize diagnosis, prognosis, and even treatment. AI-powered algorithms are capable of analyzing tissue samples with a level of detail and accuracy that surpasses human capabilities. They can identify subtle patterns and variations within cellular structures, detect minute biomarkers that may be missed by the human eye, and provide objective insights that enhance the diagnostic process.

One of the key applications of AI in pathology is the automated identification of specific biomarkers. Biomarkers are molecules or genetic signatures that indicate the presence or progression of a disease. These markers can be proteins, enzymes, or even specific DNA sequences. By analyzing tissue samples for the presence of these biomarkers, pathologists can obtain valuable information about the nature of a disease, its stage of development, and even the potential response to specific treatments.

AI algorithms excel at analyzing large volumes of data, identifying patterns, and classifying complex information.

This ability is particularly valuable in pathology, where tissue samples can contain vast amounts of information that is often difficult for humans to decipher. AI can process these data points with remarkable speed and precision, leading to more accurate and consistent diagnoses.

For example, in the realm of breast cancer diagnosis, AI is being used to analyze tissue samples for the presence of specific biomarkers that indicate the aggressiveness of the tumor. These biomarkers can help pathologists determine the risk of metastasis, the likelihood of recurrence, and the most appropriate course of treatment. AI algorithms are also being trained to identify subtle patterns in tissue samples that are indicative of early-stage breast cancer, potentially leading to earlier detection and more effective treatment.

AI's capabilities extend beyond the realm of cancer diagnosis. It is also being used to analyze tissue samples for a wide range of diseases, including Alzheimer's disease, Parkinson's disease, and heart disease. AI algorithms can identify specific protein aggregates associated with these diseases, allowing for earlier diagnosis and potential interventions.

The use of AI in pathology is not without its challenges. One major concern is the need for large datasets to train AI algorithms effectively. Training AI models requires access to a vast collection of annotated tissue samples, which can be difficult to acquire and may vary depending on the specific disease being studied. Moreover, the interpretation of AI-generated results requires careful consideration by human pathologists, ensuring that the insights provided by AI are integrated into the overall clinical context.

Despite these challenges, the future of AI in pathology is bright. AI is poised to become an indispensable tool for pathologists, enabling more accurate diagnoses, more personalized treatments, and a better understanding of disease processes. The integration of AI into pathology workflows has the potential to enhance the efficiency and accuracy of the diagnostic process, leading to improved patient outcomes.

AI is not simply replacing human pathologists but rather augmenting their capabilities. By leveraging the power of AI, pathologists can focus on the more complex and nuanced aspects of their work, while AI algorithms handle the more routine and repetitive tasks. This collaborative approach between humans and AI is likely to drive significant advances in the field of pathology, ushering in a new era of precision and personalized medicine.

AI is transforming pathology, moving it from a field heavily reliant on subjective interpretations to one powered by objective data analysis. This transition is not without its challenges, but the potential benefits for both patients and the medical community are undeniable. By embracing the power of AI, pathology is poised to become a more efficient, accurate, and personalized field, leading to earlier diagnoses, more effective treatments, and a better understanding of diseases. The future of pathology is undoubtedly bright, marked by the collaborative efforts of humans and AI, working together to improve patient outcomes and advance the frontiers of medical science.

## Beyond Images

The realm of AI in healthcare extends far beyond analyzing images. AI's ability to delve into vast troves of patient data from electronic health records (EHRs), wearable devices, and other sources opens up a world of possibilities for identifying patterns, predicting health risks, and optimizing patient care. It's like having a digital detective meticulously combing through a mountain of clues, seeking to uncover hidden insights that can guide medical interventions and improve health outcomes.

Imagine a scenario where a patient visits their doctor with a recurring headache. In the past, diagnosing the cause of headaches could be a complex and time-consuming process involving various tests and examinations. With AI, however, a doctor can now leverage the power of data analysis to identify patterns within the patient's EHR, wearable device data, and even social media activity, which may reveal potential underlying causes.

For instance, the AI system might detect that the patient has recently started using a new medication, experienced a change in sleep patterns, or engaged in activities that could be triggering headaches. By analyzing this data alongside the patient's symptoms and medical history, the AI system can provide valuable insights to the doctor, allowing them to make a more informed diagnosis and recommend the most appropriate treatment.

Beyond diagnosing specific conditions, AI can also play a vital role in predicting potential health risks. This is achieved by leveraging machine learning algorithms to analyze vast datasets of patient information, identifying patterns that may indicate an increased susceptibility to certain diseases. For example, by analyzing EHRs and genomic data, AI algorithms can predict the risk of developing cardiovascular disease, diabetes, or even certain types of cancer. These predictions empower doctors to take proactive steps to mitigate these risks, such as recommending lifestyle changes, preventative screenings, or early interventions.

The use of wearable devices, such as smartwatches and fitness trackers, has further revolutionized the way we collect and analyze patient data. These devices constantly monitor various physiological parameters like heart rate, sleep patterns, activity levels, and even stress levels. By integrating this real-time data into AI algorithms, doctors gain a more comprehensive understanding of a patient's overall health and well-being. This allows them to detect early signs of deterioration, identify potential complications, and personalize treatment plans based on individual needs.

For instance, an AI system can analyze a patient's heart rate data from their smartwatch to identify abnormal patterns that could indicate a potential heart attack or stroke. The system can then alert the patient and their doctor, enabling swift intervention and potentially saving lives. Similarly, analyzing sleep data from wearable devices can help doctors identify sleep disorders, such as insomnia or sleep apnea, which can have a significant impact on overall health.

The application of AI in analyzing patient data has far-reaching implications for personalized healthcare. By leveraging these insights, doctors can tailor treatment plans to individual patients, taking into account their genetic makeup, medical history, lifestyle factors, and even personal preferences. This personalized approach can lead to more effective and less invasive therapies, improved treatment outcomes, and a better overall healthcare experience.

For instance, by analyzing a patient's genetic information, AI can identify specific mutations that may increase their risk of certain diseases or influence their response to specific medications. This information allows doctors to personalize treatment plans, selecting the most effective drugs and therapies for each individual. Similarly, by considering a patient's lifestyle factors, such as their diet, exercise habits, and stress levels, AI can recommend personalized interventions to promote healthy habits and prevent disease.

The possibilities for AI in healthcare are vast and continuously evolving. With ongoing advancements in machine learning and data analytics, AI is poised to play an increasingly integral role in diagnosing diseases, predicting health risks, and personalizing patient care. As we move towards a future where healthcare is driven by data and insights, AI will be a key driver of innovation, improving patient outcomes and shaping the future of medicine.

## THE HUMAN TOUCH

The power of AI in diagnosis lies not only in its ability to detect abnormalities but also in its capacity to collaborate with human expertise. This collaboration is crucial for ensuring patient safety and optimizing treatment outcomes.

Imagine a radiologist reviewing a mammogram. AI algorithms have already analyzed the image, highlighting potential areas of concern. The radiologist, armed with years of experience, can then carefully examine these areas, considering the context of the patient's medical history, family history, and overall risk factors. The AI serves as an extra pair of eyes, offering a second opinion and potentially identifying subtle patterns that might be missed by the human eye.

However, the final diagnosis still rests with the human expert. The AI-generated results act as a guide, sparking further investigation and leading to a more informed decision. This interplay between AI and human expertise ensures a balanced approach to diagnosis, leveraging the strengths of both.

The same principle applies across various medical fields. In pathology, AI can analyze tissue samples, identify specific biomarkers, and suggest potential diagnoses. This information is then reviewed by a pathologist, who brings their expertise to interpret the AI-generated results within the context of the patient's individual case.

The collaborative nature of AI extends beyond diagnosis, shaping treatment decisions and promoting patient engagement. AI systems can analyze patient data from electronic health records and wearable devices, identifying potential health risks and suggesting personalized interventions. This information empowers patients to take an active role in managing their health, making informed choices about their care.

The key to successful AI implementation lies in fostering a culture of trust and collaboration between healthcare professionals and AI technologies. Patients, too, must understand the limitations of AI and its role as a valuable tool in their healthcare journey. By embracing the potential of AI while recognizing its limitations, we can unlock the full potential of this transformative technology, creating a future where AI empowers doctors and patients alike, paving the way for a healthier tomorrow.

The collaboration between AI and human expertise is essential for ensuring patient safety and optimizing treatment outcomes. Imagine a scenario where an AI system flags a potential anomaly in a medical image. This anomaly might be a small, subtle change that a human doctor might overlook. But the AI, trained on vast amounts of data, can recognize this subtle change and alert the doctor to investigate further.

This early detection can be critical in diagnosing diseases like cancer or heart disease at an early stage, when treatment is most effective. The AI system acts as an assistant to the doctor, highlighting potential areas of concern and providing additional information to support informed decision-making.

However, the AI system is only as good as the data it is trained on. If the data is biased or incomplete, the AI might produce inaccurate or misleading results. This is where the human element comes in. Doctors, with their experience, knowledge, and understanding of the patient's individual circumstances, can interpret the AI-generated results and make informed judgments.

They can also challenge the AI system's conclusions if they suspect something is amiss. This collaborative approach ensures that the AI is used responsibly and that the patient's safety and well-being remain the top priority.

The collaboration between AI and human expertise also extends to patient engagement and personalized care. AI systems can analyze patient data from electronic health records, wearable devices, and other sources to identify potential health risks and suggest personalized interventions. This information can empower patients to take an active role in managing their health, making informed choices about their care.

For example, an AI system could analyze a patient's health data and identify a potential risk of developing diabetes. It could then recommend lifestyle changes, such as dietary modifications or increased physical activity, to mitigate this risk. The AI system can also provide patients with educational resources and support to help them make these changes.

This personalized approach to healthcare can lead to improved outcomes and increased patient satisfaction. By empowering patients with information and tools to manage their own health, AI can help create a more proactive and patient-centered healthcare system.

However, it's crucial to address the ethical concerns surrounding the use of AI in healthcare. The collection and use of patient data must be done with transparency and respect for privacy. It's also important to ensure that AI algorithms are not biased against certain groups of people.

Ultimately, the goal of AI in healthcare is to augment human capabilities, not replace human expertise. By fostering a culture of trust and collaboration between healthcare professionals and AI technologies, we can unlock the full potential of this transformative technology, creating a future where AI empowers doctors and patients alike, paving the way for a healthier tomorrow.

## TAILORING THERAPIES FOR INDIVIDUAL NEEDS

### AI-Assisted Treatment: Personalizing Healthcare

Imagine a world where your doctor knows your body better than you do. A world where your treatment plan is tailored to your unique genetic makeup, medical history, and lifestyle. This isn't science fiction; it's the reality that Artificial Intelligence (AI) is bringing to healthcare. AI is no longer a futuristic concept; it's actively shaping the way we diagnose, treat, and manage illnesses.

The power of AI lies in its ability to analyze vast amounts of data and identify intricate patterns that might escape human perception. This allows AI to create personalized treatment plans that are far more precise and effective than traditional approaches. Let's explore how AI is revolutionizing healthcare by tailoring therapies to individual needs.

One of the most exciting areas of AI-driven personalization is pharmacogenomics, the study of how an individual's genes influence their response to medications. AI algorithms can analyze a patient's genetic information, along with their medical history and lifestyle factors, to predict how they will respond to different drugs. This allows doctors to select the most effective and safest medications for each patient, minimizing the risk of adverse reactions and maximizing treatment outcomes.

For example, a patient with a particular genetic mutation may be predisposed to developing certain types of cancer. AI-powered analysis of their genetic data can identify this predisposition early on, allowing for targeted preventive measures and early detection. This proactive approach can significantly improve cancer survival rates.

Another area where AI excels in personalizing healthcare is in the management of chronic diseases, such as diabetes, heart disease, and chronic obstructive pulmonary disease (COPD). AI algorithms can analyze patient data from wearable devices, electronic health records, and other sources to identify patterns and predict potential health risks.

This information can be used to provide patients with personalized health coaching and lifestyle recommendations, empowering them to take control of their health and prevent complications.

Imagine a scenario where a diabetic patient's smart watch tracks their blood sugar levels in real-time. AI algorithms analyze this data and identify potential spikes or drops in blood sugar, alerting the patient and their doctor to adjust their medication or lifestyle choices. This personalized monitoring and intervention can help prevent dangerous fluctuations in blood sugar and improve overall health outcomes.

AI can also personalize the treatment of cancer by providing individualized insights into tumor behavior and response to therapies. AI algorithms can analyze images of tumor cells, identify specific biomarkers, and predict how the tumor is likely to respond to different treatment options. This information allows oncologists to develop more precise and effective treatment plans, maximizing the chances of successful cancer treatment.

AI is not just about analyzing data; it's also about learning and adapting. AI algorithms are constantly being refined and updated with new data and insights. This continuous learning process ensures that AI-powered treatment plans are always evolving and becoming more personalized.

As AI continues to advance, we can expect even more personalized and effective treatments to become available. AI-powered virtual assistants will help patients manage their health conditions, provide personalized health education, and connect with healthcare providers. AI-powered drug discovery will accelerate the development of new therapies, addressing unmet medical needs. AI-powered robotics will assist surgeons in performing complex procedures with greater precision, reducing complications and improving patient outcomes.

The future of healthcare is personalized, and AI is at the forefront of this revolution. By harnessing the power of AI, we can create a future where every patient receives the right treatment, at the right time, and in the right way. This personalized approach will not only improve patient outcomes but also enhance the overall quality of healthcare.

## Predicting Treatment Outcomes

Imagine a world where doctors are armed with a crystal ball, capable of predicting the effectiveness of different treatment options with remarkable accuracy. This futuristic vision is no longer a fantasy; it's becoming reality thanks to the transformative power of Artificial Intelligence (AI). AI is revolutionizing healthcare, empowering doctors to make informed decisions based on data-driven insights, leading to personalized treatment plans tailored to individual needs.

One of the most exciting applications of AI in healthcare is its ability to predict treatment outcomes. AI algorithms can analyze vast amounts of patient data, including medical history, genetic information, lifestyle factors, and even environmental influences, to create highly personalized predictive models. These models can forecast the likelihood of a particular treatment being successful for a specific individual, providing valuable information to doctors and patients alike.

Imagine a patient diagnosed with breast cancer. Traditionally, their oncologist would rely on their experience and knowledge of general treatment guidelines to recommend a course of action. However, AI can now analyze the patient's specific tumor characteristics, genetic profile, and overall health status to determine which treatment options are most likely to be effective for that individual. This personalized approach can lead to better outcomes, reducing the risk of side effects and increasing the chances of a successful recovery.

The power of AI lies in its ability to analyze vast amounts of data and identify subtle patterns that humans may miss. By sifting through millions of medical records, clinical trials, and research papers, AI algorithms can uncover previously unknown correlations between treatment strategies, patient characteristics, and outcomes. This ability to reveal hidden connections allows doctors to make more informed decisions, choosing treatments that are most likely to benefit their patients.

Let's consider another example: a patient struggling with diabetes. AI algorithms can analyze the patient's blood sugar levels, medication history, dietary patterns, and physical activity to predict the likelihood of future complications, such as diabetic retinopathy or heart disease. Armed with this information, doctors can proactively intervene, taking steps to prevent these complications and improving the patient's overall health.

AI-powered predictive models not only enhance diagnostic accuracy but also empower patients to take a more active role in their health. Patients can use AI-powered apps to track their health data, receive personalized health recommendations, and even communicate with their doctors remotely. This increased engagement can lead to better adherence to treatment plans and improved self-management of chronic conditions.

The potential benefits of AI in predicting treatment outcomes are immense. It can:

- **Improve treatment effectiveness:** By selecting the most appropriate treatments for individual patients, AI can help doctors achieve better clinical outcomes.
- **Reduce the risk of side effects:** By predicting which treatments are more likely to be tolerated by specific patients, AI can help minimize unwanted side effects.
- **Optimize resource allocation:** By identifying patients who are most likely to benefit from specific

interventions, AI can help healthcare systems allocate resources efficiently.

- **Empower patients:** By providing patients with personalized insights into their health and treatment options, AI can help them become more actively involved in their care.

However, it is important to acknowledge the potential challenges and ethical considerations associated with AI-powered predictions in healthcare.

- **Data privacy and security:** AI algorithms require access to vast amounts of sensitive patient data, raising concerns about data privacy and security. Robust safeguards must be implemented to protect patient information and ensure responsible data usage.
- **Algorithmic bias:** AI models are trained on existing datasets, which may reflect existing societal biases. This can lead to biased predictions that disproportionately disadvantage certain populations. Rigorous efforts must be undertaken to mitigate bias and ensure equitable access to AI-powered healthcare.
- **Transparency and explainability:** AI algorithms often operate as "black boxes," making it difficult to understand how they arrive at their predictions. This lack of transparency can hinder trust and make it challenging to identify and address errors. Research is ongoing to develop more transparent and explainable AI models.
- **Human-AI collaboration:** It's crucial to remember that AI is not meant to replace human doctors but rather to augment their expertise. Human judgment

and clinical experience remain essential for interpreting AI-generated predictions and making informed decisions.

Despite these challenges, the potential benefits of AI in predicting treatment outcomes are undeniable. As AI technology continues to advance, we can expect even more sophisticated predictive models to emerge, leading to a future where healthcare is truly personalized and patients receive the best possible care.

The journey towards a future where AI empowers healthcare professionals to make more informed decisions is an ongoing one. It requires ongoing research, ethical considerations, and collaborative efforts between healthcare providers, researchers, and technology developers. By working together, we can harness the power of AI to improve the lives of countless individuals and create a healthier world for all.

## AI in Drug Discovery

Drug discovery, the process of identifying and developing new medications, has traditionally been a long and arduous journey, often spanning decades. However, the emergence of Artificial Intelligence (AI) is ushering in a new era of accelerated innovation, transforming the landscape of drug discovery. AI-powered tools are proving to be invaluable in streamlining the process, from identifying potential drug targets to simulating drug interactions and accelerating clinical trials.

At the heart of this transformation lies the ability of AI to analyze massive amounts of data, identifying patterns and insights that would be impossible for humans to discern. This data encompasses a vast array of information, including genomic sequences, protein structures, chemical properties of molecules, and clinical trial data. By analyzing this data, AI can help researchers identify potential drug targets, molecules that play a critical role in disease development, with unprecedented accuracy and speed.

One of the most promising applications of AI in drug discovery is in the identification of new drug targets.

Traditionally, this process relied heavily on trial and error, with researchers screening vast libraries of molecules to find those that interact with a particular target. However, AI algorithms, trained on vast datasets of biological information, can now predict potential drug targets with remarkable precision. These algorithms can analyze protein structures, identify key binding sites, and suggest molecules that are likely to bind to and modulate the target's activity. This accelerates the process of target identification, allowing researchers to focus on the most promising candidates, significantly reducing the time and resources required for drug discovery.

Beyond identifying targets, AI is also revolutionizing the process of simulating drug interactions. AI models can predict how a drug will interact with a biological system, including its absorption, distribution, metabolism, and excretion. This information is crucial for understanding the potential efficacy and safety of a drug candidate.

Traditionally, these simulations were conducted using complex mathematical models, which were time-consuming and often limited in their accuracy. However, AI models, trained on massive datasets of drug interactions and biological information, can now simulate drug interactions with unprecedented speed and precision.

The ability of AI to simulate drug interactions is particularly valuable in the early stages of drug discovery. By simulating the interactions of potential drug candidates with biological systems, researchers can identify promising candidates early on, reducing the number of experiments required and accelerating the overall drug discovery process. This not only speeds up the development of new drugs but also reduces the cost of drug discovery, ultimately benefiting patients.

The use of AI in drug discovery extends beyond identifying targets and simulating interactions. AI is also playing a crucial role in accelerating the clinical trial process, the final stage of drug development. Clinical trials involve testing new drugs in human subjects to evaluate their safety and efficacy. Traditionally, this process was slow and expensive, often taking years to complete. However, AI is revolutionizing clinical trial design, recruitment, and analysis, speeding up the process and making it more efficient.

AI algorithms can analyze patient data, including medical records, genetic information, and lifestyle factors, to identify suitable candidates for clinical trials. This allows researchers to recruit patients more efficiently, ensuring that the trials are well-powered and representative of the target population. AI can also help in the design of clinical trials, ensuring that the trials are optimized to collect the most relevant data and provide meaningful results.

Once the clinical trial data has been collected, AI algorithms can analyze it to identify patterns and trends, helping researchers understand the efficacy and safety of the drug candidate. This analysis can identify potential side effects, optimize drug dosage, and predict the effectiveness of the drug in different patient groups.

Beyond streamlining the clinical trial process, AI can also help researchers interpret the results of clinical trials, providing valuable insights into the mechanisms of action of new drugs and their potential applications. This information can be used to develop new drugs with improved efficacy and reduced side effects.

However, it is important to acknowledge that AI is not a magic bullet for drug discovery. While AI tools are proving to be invaluable in accelerating the process, human expertise remains crucial. AI algorithms are powerful tools but they need to be guided by the experience and knowledge of human researchers. The combination of human intelligence and AI technology is key to unlocking the full potential of AI in drug discovery.

The ethical considerations of using AI in drug discovery are also paramount. As AI algorithms become increasingly sophisticated, it is important to ensure that they are used responsibly and ethically. This includes addressing concerns about bias in algorithms, ensuring data privacy, and promoting transparency in the use of AI in drug discovery.

The integration of AI in drug discovery is already having a profound impact on the healthcare landscape, accelerating the development of new medications and therapies. As AI technology continues to evolve, we can expect even more transformative applications in drug discovery, leading to the development of personalized medications, faster treatment times, and improved patient outcomes.

This transformative potential is evident in numerous real-world examples. For instance, companies like Atomwise and Exscientia are using AI to identify potential drug targets and design new drug candidates. Atomwise, which uses deep learning to predict how molecules will interact with proteins, has successfully identified drug candidates for a variety of diseases, including cancer and Alzheimer's disease.

Exscientia, on the other hand, utilizes AI to automate the entire drug discovery process, from target identification to lead optimization, significantly reducing the time and cost of developing new drugs.

These are just a few examples of the growing number of companies using AI to revolutionize drug discovery. The use of AI in drug discovery is becoming increasingly common, and its impact is already being felt in the development of new therapies for a wide range of diseases.

The future of drug discovery is inextricably linked to AI. As AI algorithms continue to evolve and become more sophisticated, we can expect even more transformative applications in this field. From personalized medicine to the development of novel therapies, AI has the potential to revolutionize drug discovery, leading to a future where diseases are treated more effectively, efficiently, and safely.

However, this transformative potential comes with responsibilities. We must ensure that AI is used ethically and responsibly, addressing concerns about bias, data privacy, and transparency. By doing so, we can harness the power of AI to accelerate the development of new drugs and therapies, ultimately improving the lives of millions of people around the world.

## ROBOTICS AND SURGERY

The operating room has always been a place of precision and skill, but AI is poised to revolutionize the surgical landscape, ushering in an era of even greater accuracy, safety, and efficiency. Imagine a future where robotic arms, guided by sophisticated algorithms, assist surgeons in performing intricate procedures with unwavering steadiness, reducing human error and minimizing tissue damage. This vision, once confined to science fiction, is rapidly becoming reality.

One of the most compelling aspects of AI-powered robotics in surgery is their ability to enable minimally invasive procedures. Traditional open-heart surgery, for example, often required large incisions, leading to prolonged recovery times and increased risk of complications. Now, with the aid of robotic arms equipped with miniature cameras and surgical instruments, surgeons can perform delicate operations through small incisions, significantly reducing trauma to the body. This translates to faster recovery, less pain, and a quicker return to normal activities.

The precision offered by AI-powered robotics is another game-changer. These robotic systems can execute intricate movements with submillimeter accuracy, far exceeding the capabilities of the human hand. In neurosurgery, where even the slightest tremor can have devastating consequences, robotic assistance allows surgeons to operate with a level of precision previously unattainable. This enhanced accuracy is not only crucial for delicate procedures but also for reducing the risk of complications and improving overall surgical outcomes.

Beyond its role in minimally invasive procedures, AI is transforming the way surgeons plan and execute operations. Image-guided surgery, powered by AI algorithms, allows surgeons to visualize anatomical structures in real time, providing a 3D map of the surgical field. This enables them to navigate complex anatomy with greater confidence, avoiding vital structures and minimizing the risk of unintended damage.

The application of AI extends beyond the operating room itself. AI-powered systems are now being used to analyze patient data and identify factors that increase the risk of surgical complications. This allows surgeons to take proactive measures, such as adjusting medication levels or implementing specific protocols, to mitigate potential risks and improve patient safety.

Furthermore, AI is playing a crucial role in the development of new surgical techniques. By simulating surgical procedures in virtual reality, researchers can experiment with different approaches and optimize surgical workflows. This allows them to refine surgical techniques, improve patient outcomes, and reduce the need for costly and time-consuming clinical trials.

However, the integration of AI into surgery raises important ethical considerations. Concerns about the role of humans in the operating room, the potential for algorithmic bias, and the need for robust cybersecurity measures are paramount. It is crucial to ensure that AI systems are developed and implemented responsibly, prioritizing patient safety and well-being.

As AI continues to advance, its impact on surgery is likely to become even more profound. We can expect to see the development of more sophisticated robotic systems, capable of performing even more complex procedures with greater autonomy. The integration of AI into surgical training will also become increasingly important, equipping future surgeons with the skills and knowledge to navigate this evolving landscape.

The future of surgery lies in a harmonious collaboration between human surgeons and AI-powered systems. AI will not replace surgeons; it will augment their capabilities, enabling them to perform procedures with greater precision, safety, and efficiency. Together, they will usher in a new era of surgical excellence, transforming the lives of patients around the world.

## BEYOND TREATMENT

Beyond the realm of diagnosis and treatment, AI is poised to revolutionize the way we manage our health and well-being.

It's not just about treating diseases when they arise; it's about empowering individuals to proactively manage their health and prevent illnesses from developing in the first place. This is where AI's potential truly shines.

Imagine a world where individuals are no longer passive recipients of healthcare but active participants in managing their health journey. This is the vision of AI-powered health management, where personalized insights, predictive analytics, and proactive interventions become the norm. Let's explore how AI is transforming the landscape of chronic disease management, personalized health coaching, and preventive healthcare.

### 3.5.1: AI for Chronic Disease Management: A New Era of Proactive Care

Chronic diseases, such as diabetes, heart disease, and arthritis, pose a significant burden on individuals and healthcare systems worldwide. They often require ongoing management, medication adherence, and lifestyle modifications. AI is emerging as a powerful tool to support individuals in managing these conditions effectively.

- **Personalized Treatment Plans:** AI can analyze vast amounts of patient data, including medical history, genetic information, lifestyle factors, and real-time health data from wearable devices, to create customized treatment plans for each individual. These plans might include medication adjustments, exercise recommendations, dietary modifications, and other interventions tailored to the patient's unique needs.
- **Predictive Analytics and Early Intervention:** AI can analyze patterns in patient data to predict potential complications or exacerbations of chronic diseases. This enables healthcare providers to intervene early, preventing severe health events and improving long-term outcomes. For example, AI algorithms can predict the risk of diabetic foot ulcers or heart attacks, allowing for timely interventions such as foot exams or medication changes.
- **Medication Adherence Support:** Non-adherence to medications is a significant challenge in chronic disease management. AI-powered systems can remind patients to take their medications, track their adherence, and even detect potential drug interactions or side effects.
- **Remote Monitoring and Virtual Care:** AI-powered wearable devices and remote monitoring systems enable healthcare providers to track a patient's health status remotely, providing continuous support and intervention when necessary. This is particularly beneficial for individuals with chronic conditions who require frequent monitoring but may face challenges accessing traditional healthcare settings.

## 3.5.2: Personalized Health Coaching: Empowering Individuals with Knowledge

AI is ushering in a new era of personalized health coaching, providing individuals with the knowledge and tools to make informed decisions about their health. This involves not only providing information but also offering guidance and support to motivate and empower individuals to make positive lifestyle changes.

- **AI-Powered Health Coaches:** AI chatbots and virtual assistants can provide personalized health advice, answer questions, and offer encouragement based on a user's health goals and preferences. They can track progress, provide feedback, and even connect users with healthcare professionals when necessary.
- **Personalized Nutrition and Fitness Recommendations:** AI can analyze an individual's dietary habits, physical activity levels, and genetic information to provide tailored nutrition and fitness recommendations. This can help individuals make healthier food choices and develop customized exercise plans based on their needs and goals.
- **Behavioral Change Support:** AI can provide behavioral support for individuals seeking to make positive lifestyle changes. It can track patterns, identify triggers, and provide strategies to overcome challenges associated with healthy habits. This might involve setting reminders, providing motivational messages, and even connecting users with support groups.

### 3.5.3: AI for Preventive Healthcare: Catching Health Issues Before They Arise

The concept of preventive healthcare is shifting from a reactive approach to a proactive one, aiming to prevent diseases from developing in the first place. AI plays a crucial role in enabling this shift by identifying individuals at risk, promoting healthy behaviors, and facilitating early interventions.

- **Risk Prediction and Early Detection:** AI can analyze patient data, including genetic information, family history, lifestyle factors, and medical records, to identify individuals at higher risk for developing specific diseases. This allows for targeted interventions and screenings, potentially preventing or delaying the onset of serious health problems.
- **Health Promotion and Lifestyle Education:** AI-powered platforms can provide individuals with personalized information and resources on healthy habits, disease prevention, and early detection strategies. This might involve delivering tailored messages based on a user's age, gender, health history, and lifestyle factors.
- **AI-Assisted Screening and Diagnostics:** AI can analyze medical images, such as mammograms, retinal scans, and skin biopsies, to identify early signs of disease. This enables faster and more accurate diagnoses, facilitating timely interventions and improving treatment outcomes.

### 3.5.4: Real-World Examples of AI in Health Management

The applications of AI in health management are already transforming the lives of countless individuals. Here are a few examples:

- **Diabetes Management:** AI-powered platforms are helping individuals with diabetes manage their blood sugar levels, track their medication adherence, and receive personalized recommendations for diet and exercise. For example, the company Tidepool uses AI to analyze data from continuous glucose monitors and provides insights to help users make better decisions about their diabetes management.
- **Heart Health Monitoring:** AI algorithms are being used to analyze data from wearable devices to identify individuals at risk for heart attacks and strokes. This enables early intervention and potentially prevents serious health events. Companies like Cardiogram and AliveCor are leading the way in using AI for heart health monitoring.
- **Mental Health Support:** AI-powered chatbots are providing 24/7 support for individuals struggling with mental health issues, offering information, resources, and a safe space for self-reflection and emotional processing. Platforms like Woebot and Youper are leveraging AI to improve mental health outcomes.

## 3.5.5: Challenges and Ethical Considerations

While the potential of AI in health management is vast, there are also challenges and ethical considerations that must be addressed.

- **Data Privacy and Security:** The use of AI in health management relies heavily on patient data. Ensuring the privacy and security of this sensitive information is paramount. Robust data security protocols and ethical guidelines are essential to protect patient confidentiality and prevent misuse.
- **Algorithmic Bias:** AI algorithms are trained on data, and if the data is biased, the algorithms may perpetuate those biases. This could lead to unequal access to healthcare or inaccurate diagnoses for certain groups of individuals. It's critical to develop AI systems that are fair, unbiased, and equitable.
- **Transparency and Explainability:** It's important to understand how AI algorithms make decisions, particularly in healthcare where lives are at stake. Developing transparent and explainable AI systems is crucial for building trust and ensuring accountability.
- **The Human Element:** AI should not replace human healthcare professionals, but rather augment their capabilities. It's important to strike a balance between AI-powered tools and the essential human connection in healthcare.

### 3.5.6: The Future of AI in Health Management

The future of AI in health management is brimming with potential. We can expect to see:

- **More Sophisticated AI Algorithms:** Advancements in deep learning and machine learning will lead to more accurate and personalized AI-powered health management systems.

- **Integration with Wearables and Other Devices:** AI will seamlessly integrate with wearable devices, smart home technology, and other connected health platforms, providing a holistic view of an individual's health and well-being.
- **Enhanced Health Coaching and Support:** AI-powered health coaches will become even more personalized and adaptive, offering tailored advice, support, and motivation to help individuals achieve their health goals.
- **Proactive Disease Prevention:** AI will play a more prominent role in preventing diseases before they develop, leading to healthier populations and lower healthcare costs.

## Conclusion

AI is fundamentally changing how we approach health management. It empowers individuals to take an active role in their well-being, offering personalized insights, proactive interventions, and support for healthy lifestyle choices. As AI technology continues to advance, we can anticipate a future where AI plays an increasingly important role in managing chronic diseases, promoting preventive healthcare, and creating a healthier world for everyone.

CHAPTER 3

---

# AI IN THE OPERATING ROOM

## A NEW FRONTIER ROBOTIC ASSISTANCE

## ROBOTIC ASSISTANCE

The operating room, once a domain solely defined by the precision of a human surgeon's hand, is now being reshaped by the growing influence of artificial intelligence. The integration of AI-powered robots into surgical procedures marks a significant leap forward, bringing a new level of precision, control, and efficiency to complex operations. This revolution in surgical robotics promises to enhance the surgical experience for both surgeons and patients alike, opening doors to safer, more effective, and less invasive interventions.

Imagine a surgeon wielding a robotic arm, guided by AI algorithms, performing a delicate procedure with unmatched accuracy. This isn't science fiction; it's becoming a reality in operating rooms around the world. These AI-driven robots, equipped with advanced sensors and sophisticated algorithms, amplify the surgeon's capabilities, allowing them to execute intricate maneuvers with a level of precision previously unattainable. This precision is crucial in complex surgeries like neurosurgery, where even the slightest tremor can have devastating consequences.

The benefits of robotic assistance extend beyond enhanced precision. The robots themselves are designed for minimally invasive procedures, allowing surgeons to operate through small incisions. This means smaller scars, less pain, and quicker recovery times for patients. The impact on patients' lives is profound, leading to faster rehabilitation and a quicker return to everyday activities.

But the power of AI in the operating room goes beyond just physical dexterity. The real magic lies in the integration of AI algorithms into the surgical workflow. These algorithms can analyze real-time imaging data, identify critical anatomical structures, and predict potential complications before they arise. This information empowers surgeons to make informed decisions during surgery, minimizing risks and ensuring optimal outcomes.

For example, AI can analyze images from a patient's CT scan during a tumor removal surgery. The algorithm can then identify the precise location of the tumor within the surrounding tissue, allowing the surgeon to remove it with greater accuracy and minimize damage to healthy cells. This precision is particularly vital in complex cases, such as brain tumor removal, where avoiding damage to delicate neural structures is crucial.

The integration of AI in the operating room also extends to the realm of surgical planning. Surgeons can now utilize AI algorithms to simulate complex procedures pre-operatively.

These simulations allow them to refine their surgical strategy, identify potential complications, and practice the procedure in a virtual environment. This pre-operative planning enhances the surgeon's understanding of the case, leading to a more efficient and safer procedure.

The use of AI-powered robots in surgery is still in its early stages, but the potential for transforming surgical practice is immense. As AI algorithms continue to evolve, we can expect to see even more sophisticated applications in the operating room. For example, we might see AI systems that can predict the need for blood transfusions during surgery based on a patient's physiological data. This could allow surgeons to proactively address potential complications and ensure a smoother surgical experience.

Furthermore, AI could be used to develop new surgical tools and techniques. Researchers are exploring the development of miniature robots that can navigate the body's internal systems, delivering medication directly to targeted areas or performing intricate procedures with minimal invasiveness. This opens exciting possibilities for treating conditions that are currently difficult to address surgically.

The integration of AI into the surgical realm is not without its challenges. There are ethical concerns about the role of AI in decision-making, particularly in situations where human judgment is critical. The need for transparency and accountability in AI algorithms is paramount to ensure patient safety and build trust in these technologies.

Additionally, ensuring the safety and reliability of AI-powered systems in a highly critical environment like the operating room requires rigorous testing and validation.

Despite these challenges, the future of surgery seems inextricably linked to AI. The combination of human expertise and AI's computational power holds the promise of a safer, more efficient, and personalized surgical experience.

As AI algorithms continue to evolve, the line between surgeon and robot may blur, leading to a new era of collaboration and innovation in the operating room. This partnership will push the boundaries of surgical possibilities, leading to better outcomes for patients and shaping the future of medicine as we know it.

## IMAGE GUIDED SURGERY

The operating room has always been a realm of precision, skill, and meticulous attention to detail. Surgeons, armed with their knowledge and experience, navigate the intricate landscape of the human body, guiding their instruments with unwavering focus. However, the advent of artificial intelligence (AI) is ushering in a new era of surgical innovation, blurring the lines between human expertise and machine assistance. One of the most promising applications of AI in the operating room is image-guided surgery, a technology that leverages the power of computer vision to provide surgeons with unprecedented real-time insights into the surgical field.

Imagine a surgeon performing a complex procedure, their hands guided by a virtual roadmap projected onto the patient's anatomy. This roadmap, generated by AI-powered image analysis, displays the exact location of critical structures, blood vessels, and organs, helping the surgeon navigate the surgical field with greater accuracy and precision. This is the promise of image-guided surgery, a technology that is rapidly transforming the operating room, enhancing surgical outcomes, and minimizing complications.

At the heart of image-guided surgery lies the concept of real-time visualization. Unlike traditional medical imaging techniques, which produce static images, AI-powered image analysis can process images captured during surgery, generating dynamic visualizations that adapt to the evolving surgical field. This dynamic visualization provides surgeons with a constantly updated, three-dimensional view of the patient's anatomy, allowing them to see what they are operating on in real-time, even if the tissue is obscured by blood or other surgical fluids.

The key to this real-time visualization lies in the power of deep learning algorithms. These algorithms, trained on massive datasets of medical images, have learned to identify and segment anatomical structures, distinguishing them from surrounding tissues and fluids. During surgery, specialized cameras capture images of the surgical field, which are then processed by the AI system in real-time. The AI system analyzes these images, identifying critical structures, and projecting their location onto the patient's anatomy, creating a virtual roadmap for the surgeon to follow.

The benefits of image-guided surgery extend beyond simply providing a clearer view of the surgical field. By providing real-time guidance, AI-powered image analysis can help surgeons minimize the risk of damaging critical structures. For instance, in a brain surgery, AI can help surgeons avoid damaging vital blood vessels or nerves, reducing the risk of post-operative complications. Similarly, in a complex abdominal surgery, AI can assist surgeons in identifying and avoiding delicate organs, minimizing the risk of inadvertent injury.

Beyond minimizing complications, image-guided surgery can also improve surgical precision. AI-powered image analysis can help surgeons precisely position instruments and make smaller, more precise incisions. This can lead to faster recovery times, less pain, and a lower risk of infection.

The applications of image-guided surgery are vast and continue to expand. From minimally invasive surgeries, such as laparoscopic surgery, to complex procedures like neurosurgery, AI is transforming the way surgeons operate, enhancing their capabilities and improving patient outcomes.

Here are some specific examples of how AI-powered image analysis is being used to revolutionize image-guided surgery:

- **Neurosurgery:** In neurosurgery, AI-powered image analysis is being used to create detailed 3D models of the brain, highlighting key structures and blood vessels. During surgery, these models are superimposed onto the patient's anatomy, guiding the surgeon's instruments and reducing the risk of damaging critical structures.
- **Orthopedic Surgery:** In orthopedic surgery, AI is being used to analyze X-rays and CT scans, providing surgeons with a precise map of bone fractures and implant placement. During surgery, this map is projected onto the patient's anatomy, guiding the surgeon's instruments and ensuring accurate implant placement.
- **Oncology Surgery:** In oncology surgery, AI-powered image analysis is being used to identify tumors and their margins with greater accuracy. This allows

surgeons to remove tumors more effectively, reducing the risk of recurrence.

- **Robotic Surgery:** Image-guided surgery is also being integrated into robotic surgery systems. This combination allows surgeons to operate remotely, with the robot's instruments guided by real-time image analysis, providing greater precision and control.

The integration of AI into image-guided surgery is still in its early stages, but the potential benefits are undeniable. By enhancing surgical precision, reducing complications, and providing surgeons with real-time insights, AI is poised to revolutionize the operating room and improve the lives of countless patients.

While the future of image-guided surgery holds immense promise, it is not without its challenges. One key concern is the potential for algorithmic bias. AI algorithms are trained on datasets, and if these datasets are biased, the algorithms may produce biased results, leading to inaccurate diagnoses or treatment recommendations. It is therefore crucial to ensure that the datasets used to train AI algorithms are diverse and representative of the population they will serve.

Another challenge is the need for robust data security and privacy. The vast amounts of patient data collected for image-guided surgery need to be protected from unauthorized access and misuse. This requires robust security measures and strict privacy policies to ensure patient confidentiality.

Despite these challenges, the future of image-guided surgery is bright. As AI technology continues to advance, we can expect to see even more sophisticated applications emerge, further enhancing surgical precision and minimizing complications. With careful development and deployment, image-guided surgery has the potential to transform the operating room into a safer, more efficient, and more effective environment for both surgeons and patients.

## PREDICTING SURGICAL COMPLICATIONS

The operating room, once a bastion of human expertise and precision, is now witnessing the dawn of a new era, one where artificial intelligence (AI) plays a pivotal role in enhancing surgical outcomes and patient safety. AI-powered systems are transforming the surgical landscape, offering surgeons unprecedented tools to navigate complex procedures with greater accuracy, minimize risks, and optimize patient care. This chapter delves into the exciting world of AI in the operating room, exploring how AI is revolutionizing surgical practices and shaping the future of surgery.

One of the most impactful applications of AI in the operating room is the use of surgical robots guided by sophisticated algorithms. These robots, equipped with advanced sensors and actuators, provide surgeons with enhanced dexterity, precision, and control during complex procedures. Imagine a surgeon performing a delicate neurosurgical operation, guided by a robotic arm that allows for microscopic movements with unmatched accuracy. This level of precision can significantly reduce the risk of complications, leading to faster recovery times and improved outcomes. The robotic arm, trained on massive datasets of surgical procedures, learns from past experiences, adapting its movements to individual patient anatomy and surgical needs.

Beyond robotic assistance, AI is transforming the way surgeons visualize and interact with the surgical field.

Image-guided surgery, powered by AI algorithms, utilizes real-time imaging data to create three-dimensional models of the surgical area, providing surgeons with a detailed understanding of the anatomy and surrounding structures.

This technology allows surgeons to navigate complex anatomical regions with precision, avoiding damage to vital organs and nerves. Imagine a surgeon performing a minimally invasive laparoscopic procedure, guided by an AI-powered system that overlays the patient's anatomy with a real-time image of the surgical instruments, ensuring that every cut and suture is performed with pinpoint accuracy.

A crucial aspect of safe and effective surgery lies in the ability to anticipate and mitigate surgical complications. AI, with its ability to analyze vast amounts of patient data, can play a vital role in identifying patients who are at increased risk of complications. By examining a patient's medical history, genetic predispositions, and other relevant factors, AI algorithms can predict the likelihood of complications such as bleeding, infection, or delayed wound healing. This allows surgeons to take proactive measures, adjust surgical techniques, or schedule additional consultations to minimize risks and ensure the best possible outcomes for their patients.

Consider a patient scheduled for a major abdominal surgery. An AI system, trained on thousands of similar cases, analyzes the patient's medical records, identifying factors such as obesity, diabetes, and a history of smoking, which may increase the risk of postoperative complications. This early warning allows the surgeon to schedule a consultation with a nutritionist to help the patient lose weight before surgery, adjust the surgical plan to minimize blood loss, or prescribe antibiotics to reduce the risk of infection.

Beyond surgical precision and complication prediction, AI is transforming the way anesthesia is administered in the operating room. AI-powered systems monitor patient vital signs during surgery, adjusting medication levels in real time to optimize patient comfort and safety. Imagine a patient undergoing a lengthy procedure, their vital signs fluctuating constantly. An AI-powered anesthesia system monitors these changes, adjusting the dosage of anesthetic drugs to ensure a stable and comfortable experience for the patient.

The integration of AI in the operating room is not about replacing human expertise, but rather enhancing surgeon capabilities and improving patient care. AI systems are not just tools but partners, augmenting surgeon knowledge and skills, enabling them to make more informed decisions and perform procedures with greater precision and safety. The future of surgery holds exciting possibilities, where AI plays an even more significant role, automating repetitive tasks, guiding surgeons through complex procedures, and ultimately contributing to a safer and more effective surgical experience for patients.

This chapter has merely scratched the surface of the vast potential of AI in the operating room. As AI technology continues to evolve and integrate deeper into surgical workflows, we can anticipate a future where surgery becomes more precise, less invasive, and personalized to the individual patient. The journey towards this future is one of collaboration and innovation, where human expertise and AI work hand in hand to unlock new possibilities in the world of surgery.

## AI-Powered Anesthesia

The operating room, once a bastion of human expertise and precision, is now undergoing a dramatic transformation fueled by the power of AI. While robotic arms and image-guided navigation systems have already made their mark, the next frontier lies in leveraging AI to optimize anesthesia, the cornerstone of safe and comfortable surgical procedures.

Imagine a future where anesthesia is no longer a passive process, but a dynamic and personalized experience, tailored to each patient's unique needs and constantly monitored by AI. AI-powered anesthesia systems can analyze a patient's vital signs, medical history, and even real-time physiological data, providing anesthesiologists with a comprehensive understanding of their patient's state. This information empowers them to make informed decisions about medication dosages, ensuring optimal comfort and minimizing the risk of complications.

This AI-driven approach to anesthesia offers a multitude of benefits:

- **Personalized Care:** AI can analyze a patient's unique physiological characteristics, such as age, weight, and medical history, to determine the most effective anesthesia protocol. This personalized approach allows for precise medication dosages and a tailored experience, minimizing the risk of adverse effects.
- **Real-Time Monitoring:** AI-powered systems can continuously monitor a patient's vital signs, such as heart rate, blood pressure, and oxygen saturation, detecting any deviations from normal ranges. This real-time monitoring allows anesthesiologists to intervene

promptly if needed, ensuring patient safety and minimizing the risk of complications.

- **Predictive Analytics:** AI algorithms can analyze historical data to predict potential complications and identify patients at risk. This allows for proactive measures to be taken, preventing adverse events and improving patient outcomes.
- **Automated Dosage Adjustments:** AI systems can analyze a patient's response to medication and automatically adjust dosages as needed, maintaining optimal levels of anesthesia while minimizing the risk of over- or under-dosing.
- **Enhanced Patient Comfort:** By precisely managing medication dosages and monitoring patient responses, AI can help ensure a smoother and more comfortable anesthesia experience for patients.

Let's delve deeper into the mechanisms by which AI is transforming anesthesia:

## 1. Monitoring Patient Vital Signs:

AI-powered systems equipped with sophisticated sensors can continuously monitor a patient's vital signs during surgery.

These sensors capture data on heart rate, blood pressure, oxygen saturation, breathing rate, and other crucial indicators. AI algorithms analyze this data in real-time, identifying any deviations from normal ranges and alerting anesthesiologists to potential issues.

Imagine a situation where a patient's heart rate suddenly increases during surgery. This could be a sign of a critical event, such as a heart attack or a reaction to anesthesia. An AI-powered system would immediately flag this anomaly, allowing the anesthesiologist to intervene promptly and prevent a serious complication.

## 2. Adjusting Medication Levels:

AI systems can analyze a patient's response to anesthesia medication in real-time, using algorithms to adjust dosage levels as needed. This dynamic approach ensures that the patient remains comfortably anesthetized throughout the procedure, minimizing the risk of over- or under-dosing.

Imagine a patient who is receiving a general anesthetic. AI algorithms can track their brainwave activity, ensuring that they are sufficiently sedated but not excessively drowsy.

Based on these real-time analyses, the AI system can automatically adjust the dosage of the anesthetic, ensuring that the patient remains in a safe and comfortable state.

## 3. Optimizing Patient Comfort:

AI-powered anesthesia systems can also be used to optimize patient comfort during surgery. For example, AI can be used to personalize pain management protocols, tailoring medication dosages and delivery methods to each patient's individual needs.

Imagine a patient who is experiencing post-operative pain after surgery. An AI-powered system could analyze their pain levels, medical history, and response to previous medications, recommending the most effective pain management strategy. This personalized approach can significantly improve patient comfort and accelerate their recovery process.

- **Beyond the Operating Room:** The impact of AI on anesthesia extends far beyond the operating room. AI-powered systems can be used to optimize the entire anesthesia workflow, from pre-operative assessment to post-operative recovery.
- **Pre-operative Assessment:** AI can analyze a patient's medical history and identify potential risks associated with anesthesia. This information allows anesthesiologists to develop a safer and more personalized anesthesia plan, minimizing the risk of complications.
- **Post-operative Recovery:** AI can help monitor a patient's recovery from anesthesia, identifying any potential complications and recommending appropriate interventions. This proactive approach can help ensure a smoother and faster recovery process for patients.
- **The Future of AI in Anesthesia:** The future of AI in anesthesia holds immense promise for further advancements. Researchers are actively developing AI-powered systems that can.
- **Predict Patient Response to Anesthesia:** AI can analyze a patient's genetic makeup, medical history, and other factors to predict their response to different types of anesthesia. This information can help anesthesiologists choose the most effective and safest anesthetic protocol for each individual.
- **Develop Personalized Anesthesia Protocols:** AI can develop personalized anesthesia protocols based on a patient's unique characteristics and medical needs. This tailored approach can minimize the risk of complications and improve patient outcomes.

- **Automate Anesthesia Delivery:** AI-powered systems may eventually be able to automate certain aspects of anesthesia delivery, such as medication administration and vital sign monitoring. This could free up anesthesiologists to focus on more complex tasks, such as patient management and communication.
- **The Importance of Human Expertise:** While AI offers significant advancements in anesthesia, it is crucial to remember that it is a tool that complements human expertise, not a replacement for it. Anesthesiologists will continue to play a vital role in evaluating patient needs, interpreting AI-generated data, and making critical decisions.

The future of anesthesia lies in a synergistic partnership between human expertise and AI, leveraging the strengths of both to provide the best possible care for patients. AI will enhance anesthesiologists' capabilities, allowing them to provide more personalized, safer, and efficient care. As we navigate this exciting new era in anesthesia, it is essential to embrace the transformative power of AI while maintaining the core values of human compassion and patient well-being.

## The Future of Surgery

The operating room, once a bastion of human skill and precision, is undergoing a profound transformation driven by the power of artificial intelligence (AI). AI is no longer a futuristic dream; it's a reality reshaping the landscape of surgery, offering a glimpse into a future where procedures are more efficient, safer, and personalized than ever before.

The integration of AI into surgical practice is not about replacing surgeons; it's about enhancing their capabilities, augmenting their expertise, and empowering them to perform feats previously deemed impossible. Imagine a future where AI algorithms analyze patient data in real-time, identifying potential risks and guiding surgeons through complex procedures with unprecedented accuracy. This is not science fiction; it's the dawn of a new era in surgery where AI acts as a trusted partner, amplifying the human touch.

One of the most promising avenues for AI in surgery is the automation of tasks. Repetitive, intricate movements that require steady hands and unwavering focus can now be performed with the precision of AI-powered robotic systems.

These robotic arms, guided by advanced algorithms, can suture with sub-millimeter accuracy, perform delicate microsurgical procedures, and even assist in minimally invasive surgeries. By automating these tasks, surgeons can focus on the most complex and critical aspects of the operation, leading to improved outcomes and reduced risk of complications.

Beyond the automation of physical tasks, AI is revolutionizing the way surgeons perceive and interact with the surgical field. Image-guided surgery, powered by AI algorithms, allows surgeons to see beyond the visible, providing real-time visualization of anatomical structures and enhancing their understanding of the surgical environment. AI-powered systems can overlay digital anatomical models onto live surgical views, highlighting critical structures and guiding instruments with pinpoint accuracy. This technology has the potential to transform complex surgeries, reducing the risk of inadvertent damage and improving overall outcomes.

The power of AI extends beyond the operating table, playing a crucial role in predicting potential surgical complications. By analyzing vast amounts of patient data, including medical history, imaging results, and laboratory tests, AI algorithms can identify factors that increase the risk of complications.

This information empowers surgeons to take proactive measures, adjust surgical plans, and minimize potential risks before they even arise. The ability to anticipate and address potential complications is a game-changer in surgery, leading to fewer post-operative complications, shorter recovery times, and improved patient safety.

The future of surgery is not simply about automation and precision; it's about the harmonious collaboration between human expertise and AI capabilities. Surgeons, with their unparalleled experience and intuition, will continue to guide the surgical process, while AI will provide them with advanced tools and insights to enhance their decision-making and execution. This symbiotic relationship between human and machine promises a future where surgery is more personalized, efficient, and safe than ever before.

As we move forward into this exciting new era, it's essential to address the ethical considerations surrounding AI in surgery. Issues of data privacy, algorithmic bias, and the potential for unintended consequences must be carefully addressed. Robust guidelines and regulations are necessary to ensure the responsible development and deployment of AI in surgical practice. By approaching these ethical challenges with a thoughtful and collaborative approach, we can harness the power of AI to transform surgery for the benefit of all.

The future of surgery is a future where AI is not a replacement but an extension of the human surgeon's abilities. It's a future where the operating room becomes a space of enhanced precision, greater safety, and unparalleled collaboration between human and machine. This is the future of surgery, a future where the boundaries of human capability are pushed beyond what we once thought possible, leading to a new era of hope and healing.

## CHAPTER 4

---

# THE POWER OF DATA

### TRANSFORMING PATIENT CARE ELECTRONIC HEALTH RECORDS

## ELECTRONIC HEALTH RECORDS

The vast ocean of data that flows through modern healthcare systems is like a hidden treasure chest, waiting to be unlocked. Electronic health records (EHRs), those digital repositories of patient information, hold a wealth of insights that can revolutionize how we understand and treat disease. Imagine a world where AI could analyze millions of patient records to uncover hidden patterns, predict future health outcomes, and even personalize treatments based on an individual's unique profile. This is the power of AI in action, transforming the landscape of healthcare delivery and empowering us to better care for our patients.

EHRs are more than just digital versions of paper charts; they are dynamic databases that capture a patient's entire medical journey. From demographics and family history to diagnoses, medications, lab results, and even patient notes, these records provide a comprehensive picture of an individual's health.

However, the sheer volume of data can be overwhelming for human clinicians to process and analyze effectively. This is where AI steps in, offering its extraordinary ability to sift through mountains of information, identify patterns, and extract meaningful insights.

One of the most exciting applications of AI in EHR analysis is the prediction of future health outcomes. By analyzing vast datasets, AI algorithms can identify risk factors for specific diseases, predict the likelihood of complications, and even forecast the effectiveness of different treatment options. This kind of predictive analytics can empower clinicians to intervene early, personalize treatment plans, and improve overall patient care.

For example, AI could analyze the EHRs of patients with heart failure to identify individuals who are at higher risk of developing a cardiac arrhythmia. This early warning system could prompt clinicians to monitor these patients more closely, potentially preventing life-threatening events.

Similarly, AI could analyze data on patients with diabetes to predict those who are at increased risk of developing diabetic retinopathy, enabling timely referral for eye examinations and potentially preventing vision loss.

But the power of AI goes beyond predicting outcomes; it can also help us optimize healthcare delivery and reduce costs. By analyzing EHR data, AI can identify patterns in patient behavior, such as medication adherence, appointment attendance, and utilization of healthcare resources. This data can then be used to develop personalized interventions to improve patient engagement and reduce unnecessary healthcare utilization.

Imagine a system that identifies patients who are consistently missing appointments or not taking their medications as prescribed. AI could then trigger a series of automated interventions, such as sending personalized reminders, scheduling follow-up appointments, or connecting patients with a healthcare navigator to address potential barriers to care. This proactive approach could significantly improve patient outcomes and reduce healthcare costs.

The use of AI in EHR analysis also has the potential to transform clinical research. By analyzing large databases of patient records, researchers can identify patterns and trends that might otherwise go unnoticed. This can lead to the development of new hypotheses, accelerate the identification of potential drug targets, and ultimately lead to the development of more effective treatments.

For example, AI could analyze EHR data to identify a previously unknown genetic marker associated with a particular disease. This discovery could then lead to the development of a targeted therapy that specifically addresses the genetic defect, offering hope for a cure or more effective treatment.

However, harnessing the power of AI in EHR analysis comes with its own set of challenges. Data privacy and security are paramount concerns. Patient information is highly sensitive and must be protected from unauthorized access and breaches. Robust security measures and strict adherence to privacy regulations are essential to ensure the ethical and responsible use of AI in healthcare.

Another key challenge is the need for high-quality data. AI models are only as good as the data they are trained on.

Inaccurate, incomplete, or biased data can lead to flawed algorithms and potentially harmful outcomes. It is essential to ensure that EHR data is accurate, complete, and representative of the patient population to ensure the reliability and effectiveness of AI-powered solutions.

Furthermore, we must consider the ethical implications of using AI to analyze patient data. It's crucial to be mindful of potential biases in algorithms and to ensure that AI systems are developed and deployed in a way that is fair, transparent, and accountable. The goal is to use AI as a tool to improve patient care, not to create disparities or perpetuate existing inequalities.

Despite the challenges, the potential of AI to transform healthcare delivery through the analysis of EHR data is undeniable. By unlocking the hidden insights within this goldmine of information, AI can help us predict disease, personalize treatment, optimize healthcare delivery, and accelerate the pace of medical innovation. As we navigate this exciting new era in healthcare, it is crucial to embrace the power of AI responsibly, ensuring that technology serves humanity and improves the well-being of all.

## WEARABLE DEVICES

Imagine a world where your smartwatch not only tracks your steps and sleep patterns but also provides valuable insights into your overall health. This futuristic scenario is becoming a reality with the advent of wearable devices and the power of AI.

Wearable devices like smartwatches, fitness trackers, and even clothing embedded with sensors are revolutionizing healthcare by providing real-time data on our health and behavior. These devices can monitor a range of physiological parameters, including heart rate, blood pressure, sleep patterns, activity levels, and even blood glucose levels. This constant stream of data, once collected, becomes a goldmine for AI algorithms, which can analyze it to detect subtle patterns and anomalies that might otherwise go unnoticed.

The power of AI lies in its ability to analyze massive datasets and identify patterns that are often too complex for human eyes to discern. By leveraging machine learning algorithms, AI can extract meaningful insights from the data collected by wearable devices, providing personalized health recommendations and early warnings of potential health risks.

Let's explore some concrete examples of how AI is transforming healthcare with the help of wearable data:

- **Personalized Health Monitoring:** Imagine wearing a smartwatch that tracks your heart rate and blood pressure continuously. If you experience a sudden spike in these readings, an AI-powered system could automatically alert you and your doctor, potentially preventing a heart attack or stroke. This real-time monitoring can be particularly useful for people with chronic conditions like heart disease, diabetes, and asthma, allowing them to proactively manage their health and avoid complications.
- **Predictive Analytics:** AI can analyze your wearable data to predict future health risks. For example, if you have a history of high blood pressure, an AI system could analyze your heart rate and blood pressure readings over time to identify trends and predict when you might be at risk of a heart attack or stroke. This early warning system could empower you to take

proactive measures, such as adjusting your medication or lifestyle, to mitigate the risk.

- **Behavioral Insights:** Wearable devices can also provide valuable insights into your behavior patterns. AI can analyze your sleep patterns, activity levels, and even your dietary habits to identify areas for improvement. For example, if you consistently sleep less than the recommended seven hours, an AI-powered system could suggest strategies for improving your sleep quality, such as establishing a regular sleep schedule, creating a relaxing bedtime routine, and minimizing screen time before bed.

- **Medication Management:** For people with chronic conditions, managing medication can be a complex and challenging task. AI can assist with this process by analyzing data from wearable devices and electronic health records to personalize medication schedules and dosages. AI can also send reminders for medication refills, track side effects, and even provide personalized support for navigating medication challenges.

- **Mental Health Monitoring:** Wearable devices can also play a role in monitoring mental health. AI algorithms can analyze data like sleep patterns, activity levels, and even facial expressions to detect changes in behavior that might signal anxiety or depression. This information can then be used to provide early interventions and support for those struggling with mental health challenges.

- **Remote Patient Monitoring:** Wearable devices combined with AI have revolutionized remote patient monitoring, allowing healthcare professionals to track their patients' health remotely. This is particularly useful for patients with chronic conditions or who live in rural areas with limited access to healthcare facilities.

- **Beyond Individual Health:** The data collected from wearable devices has the potential to transform public health initiatives as well. By analyzing data from large populations, researchers can identify trends in health conditions and develop targeted interventions to address public health challenges. While the potential of AI and wearable devices to revolutionize healthcare is immense, it's crucial to address the ethical considerations and challenges involved.

- **Privacy Concerns:** The collection and analysis of personal health data raise significant privacy concerns. It's essential to ensure that patient data is collected and used responsibly, with appropriate safeguards to protect confidentiality and prevent unauthorized access.

- **Data Security:** Protecting sensitive health data from cyberattacks and breaches is critical. Robust cybersecurity measures and data encryption are essential to ensure the integrity and security of personal health information.

- **Algorithmic Bias:** AI algorithms are only as good as the data they are trained on. If the training data is biased, the resulting algorithms can perpetuate existing disparities and inequalities in healthcare. It's crucial to ensure that AI systems are trained on diverse datasets and rigorously tested for bias.

- **Transparency and Accountability:** It's vital to be transparent about how AI systems are being used and to establish mechanisms for accountability. Patients should have access to information about how their data is being used and the algorithms that are making decisions about their care.

- **The Human Element:** While AI has the potential to revolutionize healthcare, it's important to remember that human interaction and empathy remain essential in patient care. AI should not replace human clinicians but rather serve as a powerful tool to enhance their capabilities and improve patient outcomes.

In conclusion, the combination of wearable devices and AI holds immense promise for transforming healthcare. From personalized health monitoring and predictive analytics to remote patient monitoring and public health initiatives, the possibilities are vast. However, it's crucial to address the ethical considerations and challenges involved to ensure that AI is used responsibly and for the benefit of all. As we continue to develop and refine these technologies, the future of healthcare looks bright, with AI playing a central role in creating a healthier and more equitable world.

## PREDICTIVE ANALYTICS

Predictive analytics is a game-changer in healthcare, using the power of AI to analyze vast amounts of patient data and anticipate future health risks. This ability to peer into the future of patient health allows healthcare professionals to intervene early, implement preventive measures, and potentially avert serious health issues before they arise.

Imagine a world where doctors can identify patients at high risk for heart attacks or strokes years before they experience any symptoms. This is the promise of AI-powered predictive analytics. By analyzing a patient's medical history, genetic predisposition, lifestyle factors, and even environmental data, AI algorithms can pinpoint individuals who are at a higher risk of developing specific conditions.

For example, AI systems can analyze electronic health records (EHRs) to identify patients with a history of high blood pressure, high cholesterol, smoking, and family history of heart disease. Combining this information with data from wearable devices that track heart rate, activity levels, and sleep patterns, AI can calculate a patient's individual risk score for cardiovascular disease. This information empowers healthcare professionals to initiate preventative measures, such as recommending lifestyle changes, prescribing medications, or scheduling regular screenings.

The benefits of predictive analytics extend far beyond cardiovascular disease. AI can be used to predict the risk of developing diabetes, cancer, Alzheimer's disease, and many other conditions. Early identification of these risks allows for timely interventions, potentially preventing the onset of the disease or slowing its progression.

Here are some specific examples of how predictive analytics is being used in healthcare today:

- **Predicting hospital readmissions:** AI algorithms can analyze patient data from EHRs, discharge summaries, and social determinants of health to identify patients at high risk of being readmitted to the hospital after discharge. By flagging these patients, healthcare professionals can provide them with additional support and resources to minimize their risk of readmission.

- **Identifying patients at risk for sepsis:** Sepsis, a life-threatening condition caused by the body's response to infection, can be difficult to diagnose in its early stages. AI systems can analyze vital signs, blood tests, and other data to identify patients at risk for sepsis, enabling early intervention and potentially saving lives.
- **Predicting drug response:** AI can analyze patient genetic data to predict how individuals will respond to specific medications. This information can help doctors choose the most effective and safest drugs for each patient, minimizing adverse drug reactions and improving treatment outcomes.
- **Optimizing cancer screening:** AI can analyze mammograms, colonoscopies, and other screening tests to identify subtle abnormalities that may indicate early-stage cancer. This early detection can lead to more effective treatment and improve patient survival rates.

The potential applications of predictive analytics in healthcare are vast and continue to expand rapidly. As AI algorithms become more sophisticated and access to data grows, the ability to predict health risks will become even more accurate and impactful. However, it is crucial to address the ethical considerations surrounding the use of predictive analytics in healthcare.

Some concerns include:

- **Privacy and confidentiality:** Ensuring that patient data is used ethically and securely is paramount.

Robust data security measures are essential to prevent unauthorized access and protect patient privacy.

- **Algorithmic bias:** AI algorithms are trained on existing data, and if this data reflects biases present in society, the algorithms themselves may inherit those biases. This could lead to unfair or discriminatory outcomes for certain patient populations.
- **Transparency and explainability:** It is important to understand how AI algorithms make predictions and to be able to explain those decisions to patients and healthcare professionals. This ensures transparency and accountability in the use of AI in healthcare.

Despite these challenges, predictive analytics holds enormous promise for revolutionizing patient care. By harnessing the power of AI, we can move from a reactive healthcare system to a proactive one, anticipating health risks and empowering individuals to take control of their health. This paradigm shift will lead to earlier interventions, improved outcomes, and a healthier future for everyone.

## Personalized Medicine

Imagine a world where your doctor can predict your risk of developing certain diseases before they even manifest, or where your treatment plan is tailored to your unique genetic makeup and lifestyle. This is the promise of personalized medicine, a future where healthcare is no longer a one-size-fits-all approach but rather a personalized journey guided by the power of data and artificial intelligence (AI).

AI, with its ability to analyze vast amounts of data and identify complex patterns, is transforming the way we understand and treat diseases. It is empowering doctors to make more informed decisions, leading to more effective treatments and better outcomes for patients.

One of the most exciting applications of AI in personalized medicine is its ability to analyze patient data to identify genetic markers and other factors that influence drug response. This information can then be used to create personalized treatment plans that are more likely to be effective and have fewer side effects.

For example, let's consider a patient with breast cancer. Traditional treatment options often involve chemotherapy, radiation therapy, or surgery. However, these treatments can have significant side effects and may not be effective for all patients. Using AI to analyze patient data, including genetic information, medical history, and lifestyle factors, doctors can identify the most effective treatment options for each individual patient.

This approach can lead to a more targeted and personalized approach to cancer treatment, with the potential to improve outcomes and reduce the severity of side effects. AI can also be used to predict a patient's response to specific medications, helping doctors avoid ineffective treatments and minimize the risk of adverse reactions.

For instance, some patients may experience severe side effects from certain medications, while others may not experience any side effects at all. By analyzing patient data, AI can help doctors identify individuals who are more likely to experience adverse reactions to specific medications, allowing them to choose alternative treatments or adjust dosages accordingly.

The use of AI in personalized medicine is not limited to cancer treatment. It is also being used to personalize treatment plans for a wide range of diseases, including diabetes, heart disease, and mental health disorders. For example, AI can help doctors manage diabetes by predicting blood sugar levels, suggesting lifestyle changes, and recommending optimal dosages of insulin.

In the case of heart disease, AI can analyze patient data to identify individuals at high risk for heart attacks and strokes. This information can then be used to develop personalized treatment plans and lifestyle recommendations aimed at reducing the risk of these life-threatening events.

The benefits of AI in personalized medicine are far-reaching. It has the potential to:

- **Improve treatment outcomes:** By tailoring treatments to individual needs, AI can improve the effectiveness of therapies and reduce the risk of side effects.
- **Reduce healthcare costs:** By identifying individuals at high risk for disease and preventing unnecessary treatments, AI can help to reduce healthcare costs.
- **Enhance patient experience:** Personalized treatment plans can lead to improved patient satisfaction and better quality of life.
- **Promote preventive healthcare:** AI can help to identify individuals at risk for disease, enabling early intervention and prevention measures.

The use of AI in personalized medicine is still in its early stages, but the potential is enormous. As AI continues to evolve and more data becomes available, we can expect to see even more personalized and effective healthcare solutions.

It is important to remember that AI is a tool, and like any tool, it must be used responsibly. Ethical considerations, such as data privacy and algorithmic bias, need to be carefully addressed as AI is integrated into healthcare. It is essential to ensure that AI is used to benefit all patients, regardless of their background or socioeconomic status.

The future of medicine is personalized, and AI is leading the way. By leveraging the power of data and AI, we can create a healthcare system that is more effective, efficient, and equitable for all.

## Data Security and Privacy

The advent of AI in healthcare has brought about a paradigm shift, transforming the way we diagnose diseases, treat patients, and manage health outcomes. This revolutionary technology has unlocked unprecedented opportunities to analyze vast amounts of data, uncover hidden patterns, and personalize healthcare like never before. However, this exciting journey into the future of medicine comes with significant ethical considerations, particularly when it comes to the sensitive nature of patient information.

Data security and privacy are paramount in AI-driven healthcare, for they form the very foundation of trust between patients and the healthcare system. Imagine a world where our medical records, genetic information, and personal health data are freely accessible to anyone, vulnerable to manipulation or misuse. This scenario would not only erode patient trust but also create a chilling effect on the adoption of AI in healthcare, ultimately hindering the very progress we seek.

The immense potential of AI to improve patient outcomes hinges on our ability to safeguard sensitive data. Robust data security measures are not just ethical imperatives, but also legal requirements enforced by privacy regulations like the Health Insurance Portability and Accountability Act (HIPAA) in the United States and the General Data Protection Regulation (GDPR) in the European Union.

These regulations emphasize the importance of data minimization, limiting data collection and storage to what is strictly necessary for the intended purpose.

Protecting patient information in an era of AI requires a multifaceted approach that addresses multiple layers of security and privacy:

1. **Secure Data Storage and Access**
   - **Data Encryption:** Encryption is the cornerstone of data security, transforming sensitive information into an unreadable format, making it virtually impenetrable to unauthorized access. This applies to both data at rest, stored in databases and servers, and data in transit, being transmitted over networks.
   - **Secure Storage Infrastructure:** Implementing robust physical security measures for data centers and servers is crucial, with access control systems, surveillance cameras, and environmental monitoring to deter unauthorized entry and data breaches.

- **Access Control and Authorization:** Implementing granular access control mechanisms ensures that only authorized personnel, with specific roles and responsibilities, have access to specific patient data. This minimizes the risk of unauthorized access and potential misuse.
- **Data Masking and Tokenization:** These techniques further enhance data security by replacing sensitive information, such as patient names and social security numbers, with non-sensitive substitutes, protecting the original data from exposure.

2. **Secure Data Processing and Analysis**
   - **De-Identification and Anonymization:** To protect patient privacy during data analysis, de-identification techniques remove or modify identifying information, while anonymization strives to make data completely untraceable to individuals. This helps ensure that research and analysis are conducted without compromising patient privacy.
   - **Secure AI Model Training:** The training data used to develop and refine AI models must be carefully curated, ensuring that it does not contain sensitive information that could lead to patient identification.
   - **Privacy-Preserving Machine Learning Techniques:** Emerging techniques like federated learning and differential privacy allow AI models to be trained on distributed datasets, minimizing the need to centralize sensitive patient information.

3. **Data Governance and Compliance**

- **Data Governance Policies:** Establishing clear data governance policies and procedures ensures that data is collected, used, and managed responsibly. These policies should address data retention, data access, and data deletion guidelines.
  - **Data Security Audits:** Regular security audits by independent experts help identify and address potential vulnerabilities and ensure compliance with relevant privacy regulations.
  - **Training and Awareness:** Ensuring that all healthcare professionals and staff are adequately trained on data privacy protocols and best practices is essential to foster a culture of data security.

4. **Transparency and Patient Consent**
   - **Informed Consent:** Patients should be informed about how their data is being used, including the purpose, duration, and potential risks. They should have the right to choose whether or not to participate in data-driven research or AI-powered healthcare initiatives.
   - **Transparency in AI Systems:** Healthcare providers and developers should strive for transparency in the design and operation of AI systems, explaining to patients how AI is being used to inform their care, the limitations of these systems, and the potential risks involved.

5. **Building Trust:**
   - **Patient Empowerment:** Patients should be empowered to understand their rights and responsibilities regarding their health data, fostering a sense of control and confidence in the healthcare system.

- **Open Communication:** Fostering open communication between healthcare providers, patients, and developers is crucial to address patient concerns, build trust, and ensure responsible use of AI in healthcare.
- **Ethical Considerations:** Continuously reevaluating the ethical implications of AI in healthcare is critical, ensuring that these powerful technologies are used for good and not to the detriment of individuals or society as a whole.

Protecting patient information is not simply a technical challenge but a fundamental responsibility of all stakeholders involved in AI-driven healthcare. From healthcare providers and developers to policymakers and patients themselves, a shared commitment to data security and privacy is essential for realizing the full potential of AI in improving patient care and creating a healthier future.

## CHAPTER 5

# AI AND THE PATIENT EXPERIENCE

### ENHANCING CARE

## AI-POWERED CHATBOTS

Imagine a world where you can access medical information, get your questions answered, and schedule appointments with your doctor, all from the comfort of your own home, anytime, anywhere. This is the promise of AI-powered chatbots, a revolutionary technology transforming the way patients interact with healthcare providers.

AI chatbots are sophisticated computer programs designed to simulate human conversation, leveraging natural language processing (NLP) and machine learning to understand and respond to user queries. They are programmed with a vast knowledge base of medical information, enabling them to provide accurate and reliable answers to a wide range of health-related questions.

These chatbots can handle tasks like:

- **Providing basic medical information:** From understanding symptoms to explaining common medical conditions, chatbots can offer comprehensive explanations and guidance.
- **Answering patient queries:** Whether it's about medication dosages, side effects, or health recommendations, chatbots can provide helpful answers and support.
- **Scheduling appointments:** Chatbots can streamline the appointment scheduling process, allowing patients to book consultations with doctors, specialists, or other healthcare professionals with ease.
- **Managing appointments:** Beyond scheduling, chatbots can manage reminders, send appointment confirmations, and even provide directions to the appointment location.
- **Providing personalized advice:** Utilizing data from patient profiles and past interactions, chatbots can offer tailored advice and support based on individual needs and health histories.

The benefits of AI-powered chatbots in healthcare are numerous:

- **24/7 availability:** Unlike human healthcare professionals, chatbots are accessible round-the-clock, offering support whenever and wherever needed. This is especially valuable for patients experiencing urgent symptoms or needing information outside of regular office hours.
- **Reduced waiting times:** By streamlining appointment scheduling and providing quick answers

to patient questions, chatbots alleviate the burden on healthcare professionals and reduce wait times for in-person consultations.

- **Improved access to healthcare:** Chatbots can bridge the gap in healthcare access for underserved populations, including those living in remote areas or facing financial barriers.
- **Personalized care:** By analyzing patient data and interacting with individuals over time, chatbots can tailor their responses and recommendations to specific needs, offering a more personalized healthcare experience.
- **Reduced healthcare costs:** By providing self-service options for common inquiries and managing appointment scheduling, chatbots can free up healthcare professionals to focus on complex cases and reduce overall healthcare costs.

However, while the potential of AI chatbots is vast, it's crucial to acknowledge the limitations and ethical considerations:

- **Limited diagnostic capabilities:** While chatbots can provide basic information and guidance, they cannot replace the expertise of human healthcare professionals. They lack the ability to perform physical examinations, diagnose complex conditions, or prescribe medications.
- **Data privacy concerns:** Chatbots require access to patient data to function effectively, raising concerns about data privacy and security. Robust measures must be in place to protect patient information and prevent unauthorized access.

- **Algorithmic bias:** AI algorithms are trained on large datasets, and if these datasets contain biases, the chatbot may reflect those biases in its responses. It's essential to ensure that training data is diverse and representative to mitigate algorithmic bias.
- **Lack of emotional intelligence:** While chatbots can mimic human conversation, they lack the empathy and emotional intelligence of human healthcare professionals. They may struggle to understand and respond appropriately to sensitive or complex emotional situations.
- **Potential for over-reliance:** Patients may become overly reliant on chatbots for medical advice, neglecting the importance of seeking professional diagnosis and treatment.

The successful integration of AI-powered chatbots into the healthcare system requires a collaborative approach involving healthcare professionals, technology developers, and policymakers:

- **Healthcare professionals:** They need to be trained on using chatbots effectively and understand their capabilities and limitations. This ensures that chatbots are used as tools to enhance patient care, not replace human expertise.
- **Technology developers:** They need to develop chatbots that are ethically sound, data-secure, and designed to meet the specific needs of the healthcare system. Transparency in chatbot development is crucial to build patient trust.

- **Policymakers:** They need to establish clear guidelines and regulations for the development and deployment of AI chatbots in healthcare, addressing data privacy, ethical concerns, and ensuring patient safety.

The future of AI-powered chatbots in healthcare is promising, offering the potential to revolutionize the patient experience and improve access to healthcare. However, realizing this potential requires careful consideration of ethical implications, responsible development, and a collaborative approach to integrate these technologies into the healthcare system. As AI technology continues to evolve, we can expect even more innovative applications in healthcare, further transforming the way patients receive and experience care.

## Virtual Assistants

Imagine a world where your smartphone becomes your personal health advisor, offering tailored guidance and support throughout your wellness journey. This is the promise of AI-powered virtual assistants, a transformative technology poised to revolutionize how we manage our health and well-being. These intelligent companions go beyond simply providing information; they learn from your unique health data, offer personalized recommendations, and become active partners in your health management.

One of the most powerful aspects of AI virtual assistants lies in their ability to track your health data. These assistants can connect with your wearable devices, such as smartwatches and fitness trackers, to gather real-time insights into your activity levels, sleep patterns, heart rate, and other vital signs. They can also integrate with your electronic health records, providing a comprehensive view of your medical history, prescriptions, and lab results. By analyzing this wealth of data, virtual assistants can identify trends, detect potential health risks, and alert you to any concerning patterns in your health.

This ability to monitor your health data empowers you to take a more proactive approach to your well-being. Imagine receiving personalized alerts when your blood pressure deviates from your normal range or when your sleep quality deteriorates. AI-powered virtual assistants can provide timely reminders to take medications, track your progress toward fitness goals, and offer evidence-based advice on healthy lifestyle choices.

But the power of virtual assistants extends beyond simple data tracking. They can also provide personalized health coaching, offering customized guidance and support based on your individual needs. Imagine having a virtual coach who understands your health goals, motivates you to stay on track, and adapts to your changing needs. This personalized approach can be particularly beneficial for managing chronic conditions.

For individuals with diabetes, an AI-powered virtual assistant can help them monitor blood sugar levels, adjust insulin dosages, and track their dietary intake. It can also provide educational resources, answer questions about diabetes management, and connect them with support groups. Similarly, virtual assistants can help individuals with heart disease manage their medications, track their blood pressure and cholesterol levels, and stay on top of their follow-up appointments.

Beyond managing specific conditions, AI virtual assistants can also play a crucial role in promoting overall health and well-being. They can offer personalized recommendations for healthy eating, physical activity, and stress management techniques. They can also track your progress towards your goals, celebrate your achievements, and provide encouragement when you encounter setbacks. This constant support and guidance can help you build healthier habits and maintain a positive mindset.

The personalized health management offered by AI virtual assistants is not just a convenience; it can have a profound impact on your health outcomes. Studies have shown that people who use AI-powered virtual assistants for health management are more likely to adhere to their treatment plans, make healthier lifestyle choices, and achieve better health outcomes.

As AI technology continues to evolve, virtual assistants are becoming even more sophisticated. They are incorporating natural language processing capabilities to engage in more human-like conversations, allowing them to understand your questions and provide personalized answers. They are also integrating with other healthcare systems, such as telemedicine platforms, to provide seamless access to healthcare services.

The integration of AI into healthcare is a powerful tool that is transforming how we manage our health and well-being.

AI-powered virtual assistants are at the forefront of this transformation, offering personalized health management that empowers individuals to take control of their health and live healthier, more fulfilling lives. They are not simply tools, but rather partners in our health journey, offering support, guidance, and encouragement every step of the way. As we continue to explore the potential of AI in healthcare, virtual assistants are poised to play an increasingly important role in shaping the future of health management and well-being.

## TELEMEDICINE

Telemedicine, once a futuristic concept, is rapidly becoming a reality thanks to the transformative power of AI. This technology is bridging geographical and socioeconomic barriers, extending the reach of healthcare to underserved populations who may have limited access to medical specialists or face financial constraints. AI-powered telemedicine platforms are enabling remote consultations, facilitating diagnosis through sophisticated image analysis, and providing continuous patient monitoring—all from the comfort of a patient's home.

Imagine a scenario where a remote village in a developing country lacks access to a cardiologist. A patient experiencing chest pains would typically have to travel long distances, often with limited transportation options, to seek specialized care. However, with the advent of AI-powered telemedicine, the patient can now consult a cardiologist virtually. Through video conferencing, the doctor can assess the patient's symptoms, review their medical history, and even analyze electrocardiogram (ECG) data transmitted remotely. AI algorithms can analyze the ECG data in real-time, identifying potential abnormalities and suggesting appropriate treatment. This not only saves the patient time, effort, and financial resources but also provides access to specialist care that may have been previously unavailable.

Beyond remote consultations, AI is revolutionizing the way diagnoses are made through telemedicine. Consider a patient living in a rural area with limited access to advanced imaging facilities. With AI-powered image analysis, a radiologist located hundreds of miles away can analyze X-rays, MRIs, or CT scans transmitted from the patient's local clinic. AI algorithms can identify patterns and anomalies in these images, aiding the radiologist in making a more accurate diagnosis. This technology is particularly impactful in fields like radiology, where AI can assist radiologists in detecting early signs of cancer, heart disease, and other critical conditions.

Continuous patient monitoring is another area where AI is transforming telemedicine. Wearable devices like smartwatches and fitness trackers are becoming increasingly sophisticated, collecting data on a patient's vital signs, activity levels, and sleep patterns. AI algorithms can analyze this data in real-time, identifying potential health risks and alerting healthcare providers to any concerning changes.

This enables proactive care, allowing doctors to intervene before a condition worsens, preventing hospitalizations and improving patient outcomes.

For instance, patients with chronic conditions like diabetes can benefit greatly from AI-powered telemedicine. A wearable device can track their blood sugar levels continuously, transmitting this information to a dedicated app. AI algorithms can then analyze the data, providing personalized recommendations to the patient, such as adjusting insulin dosages or making lifestyle changes. This continuous monitoring and personalized feedback empower patients to manage their condition effectively, improving their overall health and quality of life.

The impact of AI on telemedicine extends beyond individual patient care. It is also revolutionizing healthcare systems and improving access to medical services for underserved communities. Telemedicine platforms powered by AI can be used to deliver remote medical education to healthcare professionals in remote areas, empowering them to provide more effective care.

This can also be used to train healthcare providers in developing countries, bridging the gap in medical expertise and improving overall healthcare standards.

AI-powered telemedicine is also playing a vital role in addressing the growing demand for mental healthcare services. Mental health disorders are often stigmatized, and many people struggle to access the necessary support. With telemedicine, patients can now connect with therapists and psychiatrists virtually, eliminating geographical barriers and providing access to care from the comfort of their homes.

AI-powered chatbots can also provide initial support and guidance, providing a safe and confidential space for individuals to seek help. However, the widespread adoption of AI-powered telemedicine also presents certain challenges. Concerns around data security and privacy are paramount. Ensuring that patient data is collected, stored, and used responsibly is crucial to maintain trust and protect sensitive information. Additionally, there are concerns regarding the potential for algorithmic bias, where AI models trained on biased datasets may perpetuate existing health disparities. It is essential to address these challenges through robust ethical guidelines and regulations to ensure the equitable and responsible development and deployment of AI in telemedicine.

Despite these challenges, the potential of AI to revolutionize telemedicine is undeniable. By enabling remote consultations, facilitating diagnosis, and providing continuous patient monitoring, AI is breaking down barriers to healthcare access, empowering individuals to take control of their health, and shaping the future of medicine. As AI technology continues to advance, we can expect even more innovative applications in telemedicine, further expanding healthcare reach and improving patient outcomes for all.

## Personalized Education

Imagine a world where you have access to a personalized library of health information, tailored to your specific needs and preferences. This library wouldn't be filled with bulky medical textbooks or dense scientific articles; instead, it would be a digital portal offering clear, concise, and engaging content that helps you understand your health and take an active role in your care. This is the promise of AI-powered personalized education, a transformative approach that empowers patients to become active participants in their own health journey.

AI has the potential to revolutionize the way patients learn about their health. Gone are the days of relying solely on the information provided by healthcare providers during brief office visits. With AI-powered tools, patients can access a wealth of personalized health information whenever and wherever they need it. This personalized education extends beyond just providing information; it involves tailoring the content to individual needs and learning styles, ensuring that patients understand the information and are able to apply it to their lives.

One of the most exciting aspects of AI-powered personalized education is its ability to leverage the power of data. By analyzing patient data from electronic health records, wearable devices, and other sources, AI can identify individual health risks, preferences, and learning styles. This data-driven approach enables the creation of highly personalized learning experiences that cater to each patient's unique needs.

For example, an AI-powered system could analyze a patient's medical history, medication list, and lifestyle data to identify specific health risks and tailor educational content accordingly. A patient with diabetes might receive personalized information on managing their blood sugar levels, making healthy food choices, and understanding the potential complications of the disease. This approach goes beyond general health education and provides targeted information that is most relevant to the individual.

AI can also enhance the engagement and effectiveness of health education by adapting to individual learning preferences. Some patients may prefer to learn through interactive simulations or virtual reality experiences, while others may prefer text-based materials or engaging videos.

AI can analyze patient data to identify their preferred learning styles and recommend content formats that are most likely to be effective.

Imagine a patient with a new diagnosis of breast cancer who wants to learn more about their condition and treatment options. An AI-powered education platform could analyze their preferences and offer a personalized learning pathway that includes interactive simulations of different treatment options, informative videos explaining the disease and its causes, and access to online support groups. This approach not only provides relevant information but also makes the learning process more engaging and empowering.

The benefits of personalized education extend beyond just increasing patient knowledge. It can lead to improved health outcomes, increased patient satisfaction, and enhanced healthcare efficiency. When patients are empowered with the knowledge and tools to manage their health effectively, they are more likely to adhere to treatment plans, make healthy lifestyle choices, and proactively manage their conditions.

For example, AI-powered platforms can provide patients with personalized reminders for medication refills, track their progress with exercise and diet plans, and even offer personalized coaching to help them stay motivated and engaged in their health journey. This proactive approach can help patients take control of their health and achieve better outcomes.

Personalized education can also help reduce healthcare costs by empowering patients to make informed decisions about their care. By understanding their health risks and treatment options, patients are better equipped to engage in shared decision-making with their healthcare providers, leading to more effective and less costly treatment plans.

However, the development and implementation of AI-powered personalized education must be approached with caution. It is crucial to ensure that these systems are built on ethical principles and designed to protect patient privacy and data security. It's essential to avoid perpetuating existing health inequities and ensure that all patients, regardless of their socioeconomic status, have access to personalized education.

Furthermore, the integration of AI into healthcare education requires a delicate balance between technology and the human touch. While AI can personalize learning experiences and provide access to vast amounts of information, it cannot replace the empathy, compassion, and personalized support that healthcare professionals provide.

The future of healthcare education lies in a collaborative approach where AI serves as a powerful tool to empower patients and enhance the role of healthcare professionals. By combining the strengths of technology and human expertise, we can create a healthcare system that is more patient-centered, engaging, and effective.

As we navigate the ever-evolving landscape of healthcare, AI-powered personalized education offers a transformative opportunity to empower patients to take an active role in their health journey. By embracing this exciting new frontier, we can pave the way for a future where healthcare is more accessible, personalized, and empowering for everyone.

## BUILDING TRUST

Building trust is the cornerstone of any successful healthcare relationship, and this holds even truer when AI steps into the picture. AI-powered systems are transforming healthcare, but for patients, it's a double-edged sword: the promise of faster diagnosis, tailored treatments, and proactive care is juxtaposed with the understandable anxieties about relinquishing control to machines. While the benefits are undeniable, the human element, the feeling of being understood and cared for, remains paramount. To bridge this gap, we must acknowledge and address patient concerns head-on, fostering open communication and transparency.

Imagine a patient, Ms. Jones, who is diagnosed with breast cancer. The news itself is a blow, and then the doctor informs her that an AI system analyzed her mammogram, contributing to the diagnosis. While she might be relieved by the speed and accuracy of the AI, fear and uncertainty may creep in. Questions arise: "How does this AI work?" "Is it truly reliable?" "What if it misses something?" These concerns are valid and deserve to be addressed honestly and empathetically.

Transparency is key. Healthcare professionals must be willing to explain the AI system to patients in clear, understandable terms. Instead of simply stating "AI identified the cancer," a more detailed explanation could be: "Our advanced imaging system uses AI to analyze mammograms, looking for subtle patterns that can be difficult for the human eye to detect. This AI system has been rigorously tested and has proven to be highly accurate in identifying early signs of breast cancer."

Furthermore, patients should be informed that the AI system is a tool, not a replacement for their doctor's expertise. They should be reassured that their doctor will ultimately make treatment decisions based on a comprehensive evaluation of their individual case. The AI system serves as an aid, providing valuable insights and supporting their doctor's judgment.

This transparency fosters trust and empowers patients to become active participants in their healthcare. Patients can feel confident that the AI system is not a black box but a valuable tool that enhances their care.

Communication is as vital as transparency. Patients should feel comfortable asking questions about the AI system and receiving clear, concise answers. Doctors and other healthcare professionals should be trained to communicate effectively about AI, addressing concerns and dispelling myths.

Imagine a scenario where Mr. Smith is scheduled for a surgery. He learns that a robotic surgical system guided by AI will be used during the procedure. He feels a mixture of curiosity and apprehension. He asks his surgeon: "Can you tell me more about this robotic system? How does it work?" The surgeon responds patiently: "This robotic system uses AI to enhance my precision and control during the surgery.

It's like having a second pair of hands that are guided by sophisticated algorithms. But remember, I am ultimately in charge of the surgery, and I will be closely monitoring the system throughout the procedure." This communication reassures Mr. Smith, allowing him to better understand the process and feel confident in the care he is receiving.

Building trust goes beyond mere information. It's about active listening, empathy, and understanding patients' perspectives. Healthcare professionals must be willing to acknowledge the fears and anxieties that patients may have about AI. They should listen attentively, validate their concerns, and provide reassurance that their well-being is paramount.

Let's consider Ms. Lee, who is concerned about the potential for bias in AI-driven diagnosis. She worries that the AI system might be more likely to miss certain conditions in certain demographic groups. Her doctor recognizes her concern and says: "I understand your worries, Ms. Lee. It's important to note that AI systems are developed with the goal of being fair and unbiased. However, we are constantly working to address potential biases and ensure that these systems treat all patients fairly. I want to assure you that I will be carefully reviewing the AI's findings and using my clinical judgment to make the best decisions for your care." This response acknowledges Ms. Lee's concern, reassures her about efforts to mitigate bias, and emphasizes the human element in the decision-making process.

Finally, the success of AI in healthcare hinges on patient engagement and participation. Patients need to be empowered to ask questions, share their concerns, and contribute to the development of AI systems that meet their needs. By engaging patients in the process, healthcare professionals can ensure that AI is not just a technological advancement but a true partner in improving patient care.

In conclusion, building trust between patients and AI-powered healthcare systems is a delicate yet crucial endeavor. It demands transparency, communication, empathy, and patient engagement. By fostering a culture of open dialogue, addressing concerns head-on, and empowering patients to participate in their care, healthcare professionals can pave the way for a future where AI truly enhances the human experience of healthcare.

## CHAPTER 6

─────────

# THE FUTURE OF AI IN HEALTHCARE

### A GLIMPSE INTO TOMORROW

## ADVANCEMENTS IN DEEP LEARNING

Deep learning, a subset of machine learning, has emerged as a transformative force in AI, particularly in healthcare. Its ability to analyze complex patterns, learn from vast amounts of data, and adapt to new information has opened up unprecedented opportunities for improving patient care. One of the most significant advancements in deep learning is the development of convolutional neural networks (CNNs).

CNNs are specifically designed to process image data, making them ideal for medical imaging applications. They can analyze X-rays, CT scans, MRIs, and other medical images to identify subtle abnormalities that may be missed by human eyes. For example, CNNs have been shown to improve the detection rate of breast cancer in mammograms, diabetic retinopathy in retinal scans, and lung cancer in chest X-rays.

Another key advancement in deep learning is the use of recurrent neural networks (RNNs) for processing sequential data.

RNNs are particularly well-suited for analyzing patient data over time, such as electronic health records, wearable device data, and medical text. They can identify patterns and trends in this data, leading to more accurate predictions of health risks, disease progression, and treatment outcomes.

The advancements in deep learning have also led to the development of new AI techniques for drug discovery and development. By analyzing large datasets of chemical compounds and biological targets, deep learning algorithms can identify potential drug candidates and predict their efficacy. This has the potential to accelerate the drug discovery process, reducing the time and cost of bringing new drugs to market.

Deep learning is also transforming the field of personalized medicine. By analyzing a patient's genetic makeup, medical history, and lifestyle factors, deep learning algorithms can create personalized treatment plans that are tailored to individual needs. This allows for more effective treatment, fewer side effects, and better overall outcomes.

The potential of deep learning in healthcare is immense. As the field continues to evolve, we can expect even more transformative applications. Here are some areas where deep learning is poised to make a major impact:

- **Early Disease Detection:** Deep learning can be used to detect diseases at earlier stages, when they are more treatable. This can lead to improved patient outcomes and reduced healthcare costs.
- **Precision Medicine:** Deep learning can help personalize treatment plans to individual patients'

needs, leading to more effective and less invasive therapies.

- **Drug Discovery and Development:** Deep learning can accelerate the discovery and development of new drugs and therapies, addressing unmet medical needs.
- **Medical Imaging Analysis:** Deep learning can improve the accuracy and speed of medical image analysis, leading to faster diagnoses and more effective treatment.
- **Patient Monitoring:** Deep learning can be used to analyze patient data from wearable devices and other sources, providing real-time insights into patient health and identifying potential complications.

## Healthcare Administration

Deep learning can optimize healthcare operations, improving efficiency, reducing costs, and enhancing patient satisfaction.

However, the use of deep learning in healthcare also presents challenges. One key concern is the need for large, high-quality datasets to train these algorithms. Acquiring and labeling such data can be time-consuming and expensive.

Another challenge is the interpretability of deep learning models. While these models can achieve high accuracy, it can be difficult to understand how they arrive at their predictions. This lack of transparency can make it difficult to trust these models in healthcare settings.

Despite these challenges, deep learning has the potential to revolutionize healthcare. As the field continues to develop, we can expect even more innovative applications that will improve patient care and enhance the healthcare system as a whole.

In conclusion, deep learning is a powerful tool that is transforming the healthcare landscape. By analyzing complex data and identifying subtle patterns, deep learning algorithms are improving diagnosis, personalizing treatment, accelerating drug discovery, and enhancing the patient experience. As deep learning continues to advance, its impact on healthcare will only grow, leading to a future of more accurate diagnoses, personalized care, and healthier lives.

## AI for Drug Discovery

The journey to discover and develop new drugs and therapies has historically been a long and arduous one.

Traditional drug discovery methods often involve painstaking research, lengthy clinical trials, and significant financial investment. However, the advent of artificial intelligence (AI) is ushering in a new era of innovation, promising to accelerate this process and potentially revolutionize the way we treat diseases.

AI's ability to analyze vast amounts of data and identify complex patterns is proving to be a game-changer in drug discovery. By leveraging machine learning algorithms, AI can sift through massive datasets of scientific literature, experimental results, and patient records to uncover previously unknown connections and potential drug targets.

One of the most exciting applications of AI in drug discovery is the identification of novel drug targets.

Traditional drug discovery often focuses on known targets, but AI can help identify new targets based on their association with disease pathways and their potential for drug development. This has the potential to unlock entirely new avenues for drug discovery and address unmet medical needs.

AI is also transforming the process of drug design. By using AI-powered tools, scientists can simulate drug interactions with target molecules, predict drug efficacy, and optimize drug properties. This allows for the rapid design and screening of potential drug candidates, significantly reducing the time and cost involved in drug development.

Furthermore, AI is playing a critical role in accelerating the clinical trial process. By analyzing patient data and identifying suitable candidates for clinical trials, AI can streamline the recruitment process and optimize trial design.

AI-powered tools can also help monitor patient outcomes and identify early signs of potential adverse events, improving the efficiency and safety of clinical trials.

The potential impact of AI on drug discovery is immense. By accelerating the discovery, design, and development of new drugs, AI has the potential to bring innovative therapies to patients faster and at a lower cost. This could lead to groundbreaking treatments for a wide range of diseases, including cancer, Alzheimer's disease, and infectious diseases.

Here are some specific examples of how AI is already making a difference in drug discovery:

- **AI-powered drug discovery platform Atomwise**, has identified potential drug candidates for several diseases, including Alzheimer's disease and cancer. Atomwise uses deep learning to analyze the structure of proteins and identify molecules that can bind to them, potentially blocking disease pathways.

- **Exscientia, a leading AI-driven pharmaceutical company**, has developed a novel drug candidate for obsessive-compulsive disorder (OCD) using AI-powered drug discovery technology. The drug candidate, called EXS-21546, is currently in clinical trials and has shown promising results.
- **BenevolentAI, an AI-focused drug discovery company**, has identified a new potential drug target for Alzheimer's disease using AI to analyze large datasets of scientific literature and clinical trial data.

The examples above highlight the potential of AI to transform drug discovery and bring new hope to patients with unmet medical needs.

While AI offers significant potential in drug discovery, it's important to recognize that it's not a magic bullet. AI-powered drug discovery requires careful consideration of ethical implications, ensuring data privacy, and validating AI predictions through traditional scientific methods.

## Beyond Drug Discovery: AI's Impact on Treatment Development and Delivery

AI's impact on healthcare extends far beyond drug discovery. AI is also revolutionizing the way we treat diseases, personalize care, and optimize healthcare delivery.

- **AI-powered Treatment Optimization:** AI is being used to personalize treatment plans based on individual patient characteristics, such as genetic makeup, medical history, and lifestyle factors. This approach, known as precision medicine, aims to optimize treatment outcomes and minimize side effects.

- **AI in Medical Imaging:** AI algorithms are being used to analyze medical images, such as X-rays, CT scans, and MRIs, to detect subtle abnormalities that human eyes may miss. This can lead to earlier diagnoses and more effective treatment.

- **AI-assisted Surgery:** AI-powered robotic systems are being used to assist surgeons in performing complex procedures with greater accuracy and precision. These systems can also provide real-time image guidance and help minimize tissue damage.

- **AI in Telemedicine:** AI is enabling remote consultations, diagnosis, and monitoring through telemedicine platforms. This expands access to healthcare for underserved populations and allows patients to receive care from the comfort of their own homes.

- **AI in Patient Monitoring:** AI-powered wearable devices and sensors are being used to monitor patient health in real-time. This data can be used to identify potential health problems early and allow for timely interventions.

The future of AI in healthcare is bright. As AI technology continues to advance, we can expect to see even more innovative applications that improve patient outcomes, reduce healthcare costs, and enhance the overall patient experience.

- **Navigating the AI Revolution in Healthcare:**
  While the potential of AI in healthcare is exciting, it's

important to navigate this revolution responsibly. Some key considerations include:

- **Ethical Considerations:** As AI systems become more integrated into healthcare, it's essential to address ethical concerns, such as data privacy, algorithmic bias, and the potential for job displacement.
- **Data Security and Privacy:** Protecting patient data is paramount. Robust security measures must be implemented to safeguard sensitive information.
- **Collaboration and Partnerships:** Successful implementation of AI in healthcare requires collaboration between healthcare professionals, researchers, and technology companies.
- **Education and Training:** Healthcare professionals need to be educated and trained on how to use AI effectively and safely.
- **Transparency and Communication:** Open communication about AI's role in healthcare is crucial to build trust and ensure patient acceptance.

The AI revolution in healthcare is underway. By embracing innovation, addressing ethical concerns, and working together, we can harness the power of AI to create a healthier future for everyone.

## Personalized Healthcare

The future of personalized medicine, driven by AI, holds the promise of revolutionizing healthcare by tailoring treatment plans to individual patients' needs and genetic profiles.

Imagine a world where doctors can predict with accuracy how a patient will respond to a specific medication based on their unique genetic makeup, eliminating trial-and-error approaches and minimizing side effects. This is the potential of personalized medicine, powered by AI.

The core of personalized medicine lies in understanding an individual's unique genetic blueprint. Through advanced genetic sequencing and analysis, AI algorithms can decipher the intricate code of a patient's DNA, identifying specific genetic markers that influence disease susceptibility, drug response, and even treatment outcomes. This information, combined with a comprehensive understanding of a patient's medical history, lifestyle factors, and environmental exposures, allows AI to create highly personalized treatment plans that are optimized for each individual.

AI-powered personalized medicine goes beyond simply identifying genetic variations; it delves into the complex interplay between genes and the environment. AI algorithms can analyze vast datasets of patient information, including genetic data, medical records, lifestyle choices, and environmental factors, to identify intricate patterns and correlations that might otherwise go unnoticed. This ability to uncover hidden relationships between genetic predisposition, lifestyle choices, and disease development allows for a more holistic understanding of an individual's health and the development of personalized strategies for prevention, early detection, and targeted treatment.

The impact of AI-powered personalized medicine on various medical fields is profound. In oncology, for instance, AI can analyze tumor biopsies and genetic profiles to identify the specific genetic mutations driving cancer growth. This information can then guide the selection of targeted therapies that effectively attack the cancerous cells while minimizing damage to healthy tissues. Similarly, in cardiology, AI can analyze a patient's genetic profile and lifestyle factors to assess their risk for cardiovascular disease and tailor preventive strategies accordingly.

AI-powered personalized medicine also promises to revolutionize drug discovery and development. By analyzing massive datasets of molecular structures and biological pathways, AI algorithms can identify potential drug targets and predict their effectiveness in treating specific diseases.

This can significantly accelerate the drug development process, reducing the time and cost associated with traditional methods. Furthermore, AI can help predict how different drugs might interact with a patient's individual genetic makeup, minimizing the risk of adverse drug reactions and ensuring optimal treatment outcomes.

Beyond its application in individual patient care, AI-powered personalized medicine also has the potential to transform public health strategies. By analyzing large datasets of patient information, AI algorithms can identify emerging disease trends, predict outbreaks, and even develop tailored public health interventions to address specific health concerns within different populations. This can lead to more effective and efficient disease prevention and control strategies, ultimately contributing to a healthier society.

While the potential of AI-powered personalized medicine is enormous, it is crucial to address the ethical considerations and challenges associated with its implementation. One key concern is the potential for genetic discrimination, where individuals may be denied insurance or employment opportunities based on their genetic predisposition to certain diseases. Ensuring data privacy and security is another critical concern, as vast amounts of sensitive patient data will be analyzed and used for personalized treatment plans.

Furthermore, the development and deployment of AI-powered personalized medicine must be transparent and inclusive. It is crucial to involve patients in the decision-making process regarding the use of their genetic information and ensure that they have access to clear and understandable information about how AI is being used to personalize their care. It is equally important to ensure that AI systems are developed and deployed in a fair and equitable manner, addressing potential biases that could disproportionately impact certain populations.

The future of personalized medicine is bright, with AI poised to revolutionize healthcare by tailoring treatment plans to individual needs. However, it is essential to proceed with caution, addressing the ethical and societal implications of this transformative technology to ensure that it is used responsibly and equitably for the benefit of all. As we navigate the exciting but complex landscape of AI-powered personalized medicine, collaboration between healthcare professionals, researchers, policymakers, and patients is essential to realize the full potential of this transformative technology and create a healthier future for all.

## AI AND THE HUMAN CONNECTION

The future of healthcare, as envisioned by the integration of AI, paints a vibrant picture of a symbiotic relationship between human expertise and intelligent machines. Imagine a world where doctors are not just diagnosing and treating diseases but also collaborating with AI partners to unlock deeper insights, predict potential complications with unparalleled accuracy, and personalize treatment plans that cater to each patient's unique needs. This isn't science fiction; it's the reality we're rapidly approaching.

AI, in this future, acts as an extension of human capabilities, amplifying their knowledge and skills. It doesn't replace human doctors; it empowers them, allowing them to focus on what matters most: the human touch, empathy, and the nuances of individual patient experiences. Imagine a radiologist, not burdened by tedious tasks of analyzing countless images, but instead, assisted by AI that highlights areas of concern, enabling the doctor to focus on making crucial diagnoses with greater precision. This partnership between human expertise and AI's analytical power represents a paradigm shift in healthcare, leading to earlier diagnoses, more effective treatments, and ultimately, better patient outcomes.

One of the most exciting areas of collaboration between AI and healthcare professionals lies in the field of predictive analytics. AI algorithms, trained on vast datasets of patient information, can identify patterns and predict potential health risks with remarkable accuracy. This allows doctors to proactively intervene and prevent disease progression.

Imagine a patient with a family history of heart disease. By analyzing the patient's genetic data, lifestyle choices, and medical history, AI can predict their risk of developing heart disease and recommend preventative measures like lifestyle changes, personalized medication, or even early screening tests. This proactive approach can dramatically improve patient outcomes and reduce the burden of chronic diseases.

The power of AI doesn't stop at diagnosis and prevention; it extends to the realm of treatment. AI can analyze a patient's genetic makeup and medical history to personalize treatment plans, ensuring the best possible outcome for each individual. In oncology, for instance, AI can analyze a tumor's specific genetic mutations to determine the most effective chemotherapy regimen, significantly increasing treatment success rates and reducing side effects. Imagine a world where chemotherapy is no longer a grueling one-size-fits-all approach but a tailored therapy, designed to target the specific needs of each cancer patient.

But AI's impact on healthcare extends far beyond individual patient care. It has the potential to revolutionize drug discovery and development, significantly accelerating the process of bringing new treatments to market. AI can sift through vast databases of chemical compounds, identify promising drug candidates, and simulate their interactions with specific disease targets. This process, which traditionally took years, can be significantly shortened by AI, leading to the faster development of life-saving medications.

The future of AI in healthcare is not just about technology; it's about a fundamental shift in our approach to healthcare delivery. It's about embracing a collaborative model, where humans and machines work together to deliver the best possible care for every patient. This collaboration requires a shared understanding of each other's strengths and limitations, a willingness to learn and adapt, and a commitment to building trust between humans and AI.

To fully realize the potential of AI in healthcare, we need to address the ethical and societal implications of this transformative technology. Ensuring data privacy and security is paramount, as is mitigating potential biases in algorithms. Transparent communication about how AI is used in healthcare is essential to building public trust and fostering informed decision-making.

The future of healthcare, as envisioned by the integration of AI, is a future where technology empowers humans, where knowledge is amplified, and where individual needs are met with unprecedented precision and care. It's a future where the human touch remains central, but where AI acts as a powerful ally, helping us unlock the full potential of medicine to improve the health and well-being of everyone.

## A Vision for the Future

The journey towards a healthier tomorrow is not merely about advancements in medical technology, but also about how we leverage those advancements to build a more equitable and accessible healthcare system. The future we envision is one where AI, working in concert with human expertise, becomes an integral part of our lives, empowering individuals to take control of their health and access the care they need.

Imagine a world where AI-powered virtual assistants are the first line of defense against illness. These assistants, seamlessly integrated into our daily lives, monitor our health through wearable devices and analyze our personal data to detect early signs of disease. They provide personalized health coaching, nudging us toward healthier habits and reminding us of important appointments. If needed, they can connect us with healthcare professionals, ensuring we receive timely and appropriate care.

The future of healthcare is one where AI plays a pivotal role in drug discovery and development. Imagine a world where AI algorithms can analyze vast datasets, identifying potential drug targets and simulating drug interactions with unprecedented accuracy. This would accelerate the development of new therapies, leading to faster treatments for diseases that have plagued humanity for generations.

Personalized medicine, powered by AI, will revolutionize the way we treat diseases. Imagine a world where AI analyzes an individual's genetic makeup, medical history, and lifestyle factors to tailor treatment plans that are specific to their unique needs. This personalized approach would improve treatment outcomes, reduce side effects, and enhance overall well-being.

The power of AI extends beyond diagnosis and treatment; it can also help us manage chronic conditions. Imagine a world where AI-powered systems monitor patients with diabetes, heart disease, or other chronic conditions in real-time, providing personalized insights and guidance. These systems could detect early signs of complications, preventing unnecessary hospitalizations and improving quality of life for millions.

However, the future of AI in healthcare is not solely reliant on technological advancements. It requires a collective effort to ensure that AI is developed and deployed ethically and responsibly. We must address concerns about data privacy, algorithmic bias, and the potential for AI to exacerbate existing healthcare disparities.

Transparency and communication are paramount. Patients must understand how AI is used in their care, and healthcare professionals must be trained to effectively integrate AI into their practice. Open dialogue between patients, healthcare providers, researchers, and policymakers is essential to navigate the challenges and opportunities that lie ahead.

The future of healthcare is not a dystopian fantasy, but a hopeful vision of a world where AI empowers individuals to live healthier, more fulfilling lives. It is a vision of a future where technology complements human expertise, creating a more equitable, accessible, and effective healthcare system for all. It is a future where healthcare is personalized, proactive, and ultimately, more human.

The journey toward this future will require ongoing innovation, collaboration, and a commitment to ethical development. We must embrace the transformative potential of AI while acknowledging its limitations and ensuring it serves humanity's best interests. By working together, we can build a future where AI shapes a healthier tomorrow for all.

CHAPTER 7

---

# NAVIGATING THE AI REVOLUTION

## A GUIDE FOR THE FUTURE

## EMBRACING CHANGE

The winds of change are blowing through the healthcare landscape, and at the heart of this transformation lies Artificial Intelligence (AI). The AI revolution is not a distant future; it is unfolding right now, bringing about a paradigm shift in how we diagnose, treat, and manage diseases. We stand at a crossroads, where embracing AI becomes not merely a choice but a necessity to unlock a future of personalized, data-driven, and ultimately, healthier lives.

This paradigm shift demands a fundamental shift in our thinking. Gone are the days of relying solely on intuition and experience. The future of healthcare lies in embracing a collaborative approach, where human expertise blends seamlessly with the power of AI. This fusion of intelligence opens doors to unprecedented possibilities, but it also requires a commitment to continuous learning and adaptation.

Just as the medical profession has always been at the forefront of scientific advancements, so too must it adapt to the burgeoning AI revolution. Healthcare professionals must actively seek out opportunities to familiarize themselves with the latest AI technologies and explore their potential applications in their respective fields. Workshops, conferences, and online courses are becoming increasingly accessible, providing platforms for knowledge sharing and fostering a deeper understanding of AI's capabilities.

But the imperative to learn extends beyond the medical community. Patients too, must engage in this ongoing dialogue. As AI increasingly informs decisions about diagnosis, treatment, and even preventive care, patients need to be empowered with the knowledge to ask informed questions, understand the implications of AI-driven recommendations, and actively participate in their healthcare journey. This open exchange of information fosters trust and ensures that patients remain at the heart of their own care.

The adoption of AI in healthcare is not without its challenges. Concerns about data privacy, algorithmic bias, and the potential for unintended consequences are legitimate and deserve careful consideration. However, these challenges are not insurmountable. By engaging in open dialogue, establishing ethical guidelines, and prioritizing patient well-being, we can ensure that AI is developed and deployed responsibly, promoting both innovation and safety.

The AI revolution is not merely about replacing human doctors with machines. It's about creating a synergistic partnership, where AI enhances the abilities of medical professionals, freeing them to focus on the aspects of care that require human compassion, empathy, and nuanced understanding. This partnership enables doctors to deliver more personalized and effective care, while AI acts as a powerful ally in the pursuit of better health outcomes.

The adoption of AI is not a one-time event; it is an ongoing process of evolution. As AI technology continues to advance, so too must our approach to healthcare evolve. This demands a commitment to lifelong learning, a willingness to challenge assumptions, and an openness to embracing new paradigms.

Imagine a future where doctors are equipped with AI-powered diagnostic tools that can detect subtle abnormalities, predict potential complications, and personalize treatment plans with unprecedented precision. Imagine a world where patients are empowered with AI-driven virtual assistants that monitor their health, provide personalized health coaching, and ensure they receive the right care at the right time.

This vision of the future is not just a fantasy; it is a realistic possibility if we embrace the AI revolution with open minds and unwavering commitment. We must recognize that AI is not simply a technological marvel; it is a powerful tool that holds the potential to transform healthcare for the better, empowering both doctors and patients to navigate the complexities of health and well-being in a more informed, personalized, and ultimately, healthier way.

## BUILDING A SKILLED WORKFORCE

The AI revolution is upon us, and healthcare is at the forefront of this transformative wave. While AI holds immense potential to revolutionize medical practices, its successful integration depends heavily on a skilled workforce, well-versed in the intricacies of this emerging technology. This is where education becomes paramount.

Educating healthcare professionals about AI is crucial for its seamless adoption. The medical landscape is undergoing a rapid shift, and doctors, nurses, and other specialists need to be equipped with the knowledge and skills to navigate this changing environment. Imagine a scenario where a doctor is presented with an AI-generated diagnosis, but lacks the understanding to interpret it correctly or even question its validity. This scenario highlights the critical need for a skilled workforce that can effectively utilize and interpret AI-powered tools.

The challenge lies in bridging the gap between traditional medical training and the rapidly evolving field of AI. This requires a multi-pronged approach:

- **Integrating AI into medical curricula:** Universities and medical schools need to incorporate AI concepts and applications into their core curricula. This could involve dedicated courses on AI in healthcare, workshops, and interactive learning modules. Imagine a medical student learning about the latest AI algorithms for image analysis or the use of AI-powered chatbots in patient communication as part of their regular coursework. Such an approach would equip future doctors with the necessary skills to confidently utilize AI in their practice from the very start.
- **Providing ongoing professional development:** For practicing healthcare professionals, ongoing education and training programs are crucial to keep them abreast of the latest AI advancements. Workshops,

conferences, online courses, and mentorship programs can help physicians acquire the skills needed to utilize AI in their daily practice. This ensures that healthcare professionals remain relevant and equipped to handle the complexities of AI-driven healthcare.

- **Creating specialized AI roles within healthcare organizations:** As AI plays a more prominent role in healthcare, the demand for specialists with AI expertise will continue to rise. This necessitates the creation of dedicated roles such as AI specialists, data scientists, and machine learning engineers within healthcare organizations. These individuals will be responsible for developing, implementing, and maintaining AI systems, ensuring their effective integration into healthcare workflows.

Furthermore, the education of the general public is equally important. A well-informed public is essential for the successful adoption and ethical development of AI in healthcare. Imagine a scenario where patients are hesitant or even fearful of AI-driven diagnoses and treatment plans due to a lack of understanding. Addressing these concerns requires effective communication and public education initiatives.

Here are key aspects of public education:

- **Promoting AI literacy:** The public needs to be educated about the basics of AI, its potential benefits, and its limitations. Educational materials, public talks, and online resources can be used to dispel misconceptions and promote understanding. Imagine a public forum where experts discuss the role of AI in early disease detection and personalized medicine, answering questions from the audience and addressing their concerns. This kind of open dialogue fosters trust and facilitates informed discussions about AI in healthcare.

- **Addressing ethical considerations:** Open discussions on the ethical implications of AI in healthcare, such as data privacy, algorithmic bias, and potential job displacement, are essential. Public awareness about these issues ensures responsible development and deployment of AI technologies. Imagine a community gathering where researchers and ethicists discuss the ethical guidelines for using AI in healthcare, emphasizing the importance of patient consent and data security. This kind of transparent dialogue helps build public trust and ensures ethical considerations are at the forefront of AI development.

- **Empowering patients:** The public should be empowered to engage with AI-powered healthcare systems and make informed decisions about their health. This includes providing access to clear and concise information about AI-powered tools, their benefits, and their potential risks. Imagine a patient portal where individuals can access their medical records, receive personalized health recommendations based on AI analysis, and engage in virtual consultations with healthcare providers. Such initiatives empower patients to take an active role in their healthcare journey and promote a more collaborative approach between patients and AI systems.

In conclusion, building a skilled workforce and an informed public is paramount for the successful implementation of AI in healthcare. Investing in education across all levels - healthcare professionals, patients, and the general public - is crucial for ensuring a smooth transition towards an AI-driven future. By fostering a culture of understanding and knowledge, we can harness the transformative power of AI to improve patient care, enhance healthcare efficiency, and ultimately create a healthier world for all.

## PROMOTING ETHICAL DEVELOPMENT

The potential of AI in healthcare is immense, but we must tread carefully, ensuring that its development and deployment are guided by ethical principles and robust regulations. We cannot allow the pursuit of technological advancement to overshadow the fundamental values of patient safety, privacy, and fairness.

### Ethical Guidelines: A Foundation for Trust

To build trust in AI-powered healthcare, we need a clear set of ethical guidelines that govern its development and deployment. These guidelines should address the following key areas:

- **Transparency and Explainability:** AI algorithms, especially those used in critical decision-making, should be transparent and explainable. Healthcare providers and patients must understand how these algorithms work, the data they rely on, and the rationale behind their recommendations. This transparency fosters trust and accountability.
- **Algorithmic Bias:** AI systems inherit biases from the data they are trained on. It is crucial to address

potential biases that could lead to unfair or discriminatory outcomes in healthcare. Data sets used to train AI models should be diverse and representative of the population they are intended to serve.

- **Data Privacy and Security:** Patient data is highly sensitive and must be protected from unauthorized access and misuse. Robust data security measures should be in place to safeguard patient information and ensure compliance with privacy regulations like HIPAA.
- **Informed Consent:** Patients should be informed about the use of AI in their care and given the opportunity to provide informed consent. This includes understanding the potential benefits and risks associated with AI-powered systems.
- **Human Oversight:** While AI can be a powerful tool, it is essential to maintain human oversight in healthcare. AI systems should not be used to replace human judgment, but rather to augment and support clinical decision-making.
- **Accountability and Responsibility:** Clear mechanisms for accountability and responsibility should be established. In cases where AI systems make errors or contribute to adverse outcomes, there should be clear processes for identifying the cause, addressing the problem, and holding the responsible parties accountable.

## Regulation: Ensuring Responsible AI Development

Ethical guidelines provide a strong foundation, but they need to be complemented by robust regulations. Regulatory frameworks should address key aspects of AI development and deployment in healthcare:

- **Standardization and Certification:** Development and deployment of AI systems in healthcare should adhere to established standards and undergo rigorous testing and certification processes. This ensures quality, safety, and efficacy
- **Data Governance:** Clear regulations governing the collection, use, and sharing of patient data are essential. These regulations should address data privacy, security, and consent requirements.
- **Algorithmic Transparency:** Regulations should require transparency in the design and operation of AI algorithms, particularly those used in diagnosis and treatment. This includes providing documentation, access to data, and explanations for algorithmic decisions.
- **Risk Assessment and Mitigation:** Regulatory frameworks should require thorough risk assessment of AI systems, identifying potential risks and developing strategies to mitigate them. This ensures patient safety and avoids unintended consequences.
- **Monitoring and Evaluation:** Ongoing monitoring and evaluation of AI systems are crucial to ensure their continued effectiveness and safety. This includes tracking performance metrics, identifying potential issues, and adapting systems as needed.

## Collaborations for Ethical AI Development

The responsible development and deployment of AI in healthcare require a collaborative effort involving various stakeholders:

- **Healthcare Professionals:** Clinicians are at the forefront of AI implementation. They need to actively participate in the design, testing, and deployment of AI systems, ensuring they meet clinical needs and maintain patient safety.
- **Researchers and Developers:** Researchers and developers play a crucial role in advancing AI technology. They need to prioritize ethical considerations in their research and development processes, adhering to best practices and collaborating with healthcare professionals.
- **Policymakers and Regulators:** Governments and regulatory bodies have a critical role in establishing ethical guidelines and regulations that govern the use of AI in healthcare. They need to keep pace with technological advancements and ensure that regulations are effective in promoting responsible AI development.
- **Patients and Public:** Patients and the public have a right to understand how AI is being used in healthcare and to raise concerns about potential risks. Transparency and communication are essential to build trust and ensure that AI is used in a way that benefits all.

## THE ROLE OF PUBLIC AWARENESS

Public awareness is crucial in fostering ethical AI development. By educating the public about AI and its potential applications in healthcare, we can encourage informed dialogue and promote responsible innovation.

**Examples of Ethical AI Implementation in Healthcare**

Several organizations and initiatives are leading the way in promoting ethical AI in healthcare:

- **The Partnership on AI:** This non-profit organization brings together leading researchers, developers, and policymakers to discuss and address the ethical implications of AI.
- **The FDA's AI/ML Software as a Medical Device (SaMD) Framework:** The FDA has established guidelines for the development and evaluation of AI-powered medical devices, ensuring their safety and efficacy.
- **The Health Information Trust Alliance (HITRUST):** This non-profit organization provides a framework for assessing and managing data privacy and security risks in healthcare, including AI-powered systems.

## CONCLUSION

The AI revolution in healthcare presents both exciting opportunities and significant challenges. By embracing ethical development and enacting robust regulations, we can harness the transformative potential of AI while ensuring that it is used responsibly and for the benefit of all. The future of healthcare depends on our collective commitment to building an AI-powered system that is ethical, transparent, and ultimately, beneficial for patients and society.

## Fostering Innovation

The journey towards a future where AI seamlessly integrates into healthcare requires a concerted effort from all stakeholders. This necessitates fostering an ecosystem of collaboration and partnerships among healthcare professionals, researchers, and technology companies. Such collaborations are the lifeblood of innovation, driving the development of groundbreaking AI-powered tools and applications.

One crucial aspect of fostering innovation lies in bridging the gap between healthcare professionals and AI developers.

Doctors, nurses, and other medical professionals have invaluable insights into the complexities of clinical practice and the needs of patients. Their expertise is vital in guiding the development of AI tools that address real-world challenges and are tailored to the specific needs of healthcare delivery.

This collaboration can be achieved through workshops, symposia, and dedicated platforms where healthcare professionals and AI experts can engage in open dialogues, share experiences, and co-create solutions. This cross-disciplinary exchange of knowledge and perspectives is essential to ensure that AI tools are not just technically sound but also clinically relevant and patient-centered.

Furthermore, healthcare professionals should be actively involved in the evaluation and validation of AI-powered tools. This involves conducting clinical trials, assessing the performance of AI systems in real-world settings, and gathering feedback from patients and clinicians. Such rigorous evaluation is crucial to ensure that AI tools are safe, effective, and meet the highest standards of medical practice.

Researchers play a pivotal role in pushing the boundaries of AI research and development. They are the driving force behind the creation of novel algorithms, the development of new applications, and the exploration of innovative ways to harness the power of AI for healthcare. Their expertise is essential in addressing the complex scientific and technical challenges that lie at the heart of AI development.

Collaboration between researchers and healthcare professionals is crucial for translating research findings into practical clinical applications. Researchers can gain valuable insights into the challenges and opportunities of healthcare delivery from the perspective of clinicians. This collaboration can foster the development of AI tools that are not only technically sound but also practical and implementable in real-world clinical settings.

Technology companies are at the forefront of AI development, creating the tools and platforms that are shaping the future of healthcare. They have the resources, expertise, and infrastructure to develop cutting-edge AI solutions that have the potential to revolutionize medical practice. However, their efforts must be guided by the needs and priorities of the healthcare community.

Partnerships between technology companies and healthcare institutions are essential to ensure that AI development is aligned with the needs of patients and clinicians. This collaboration involves sharing data, conducting joint research projects, and developing AI tools that meet the specific requirements of healthcare delivery.

One example of a successful collaboration is the partnership between Google and the Mayo Clinic. This collaboration led to the development of a deep learning algorithm for detecting diabetic retinopathy, a leading cause of blindness. The algorithm, trained on a massive dataset of retinal images, achieved a high level of accuracy in identifying the disease, enabling early intervention and preventing vision loss.

Another example is the partnership between IBM Watson and the Cleveland Clinic. This collaboration focused on developing AI-powered systems for personalized cancer care. Watson's AI platform analyzes patient data, including medical records, genetic information, and clinical trial results, to recommend personalized treatment plans for cancer patients.

These collaborations highlight the importance of combining the expertise of healthcare professionals, researchers, and technology companies to drive innovation in AI-powered healthcare. By working together, these stakeholders can create a future where AI is a powerful force for good, improving patient outcomes, enhancing medical practice, and shaping a healthier world.

Beyond specific collaborations, the creation of a supportive ecosystem for AI innovation is crucial. This includes fostering a culture of open data sharing, promoting responsible AI development, and supporting entrepreneurship in the field of AI-powered healthcare. Open data sharing is vital for AI research and development.

Large datasets of medical images, patient records, and clinical trials are essential for training AI algorithms and developing effective AI tools. However, data sharing must be done responsibly, ensuring patient privacy and data security.

Responsible AI development requires establishing ethical guidelines and regulations to ensure that AI tools are used ethically and safely. This includes addressing concerns about bias, transparency, and accountability in AI systems. It also necessitates fostering public trust in AI by ensuring that AI tools are developed and deployed with transparency and accountability.

Finally, supporting entrepreneurship in AI-powered healthcare is crucial for driving innovation and creating new solutions. This involves providing resources, mentorship, and funding for startups and companies working on AI applications in healthcare. Such support can foster a vibrant and dynamic ecosystem of AI innovation that benefits both patients and the healthcare community.

In conclusion, fostering collaboration and partnerships between healthcare professionals, researchers, and technology companies is paramount to driving innovation in AI-powered healthcare. By working together, these stakeholders can create a future where AI is a transformative force, improving patient outcomes, enhancing medical practice, and shaping a healthier world for all.

## A Shared Future

The promise of a healthier future, where diseases are detected earlier, treatments are tailored to individual needs, and healthcare is more accessible than ever before, is a vision that AI brings into sharp focus. The transformative potential of AI in healthcare isn't just about technological advancement; it's about a paradigm shift in how we approach health and well-being.

The journey toward this shared future demands a collaborative effort. Healthcare professionals, researchers, technology companies, and policymakers must work together to ensure the ethical and responsible development and deployment of AI in healthcare. This involves:

1. **Educating the Next Generation:** We need to invest in education and training programs to equip healthcare professionals with the skills and knowledge to effectively integrate AI into their practices. This includes understanding the nuances of AI algorithms, interpreting AI-generated results, and navigating the ethical considerations involved.

2. **Fostering Collaboration:** Breaking down silos between healthcare professionals, researchers, and technology companies is crucial for driving innovation in AI-powered healthcare. Collaborative research projects, shared data platforms, and open-source initiatives can accelerate the development of cutting-edge AI solutions that address real-world challenges.

3. **Embracing Ethical Guidelines:** The development and deployment of AI in healthcare must be guided by a strong ethical framework that prioritizes patient safety, privacy, and fairness. This involves establishing clear guidelines for data privacy, algorithmic transparency, and ensuring that AI systems are designed to avoid bias and promote equity.

4. **Addressing Public Concerns:** Open dialogue and communication are essential to address public concerns about AI in healthcare. Building trust in AI-powered systems requires transparency, accessibility, and clear explanations of how AI works and how it can benefit patients.

5. **Embracing Continuous Learning:** The field of AI is constantly evolving, with new advancements emerging regularly. Staying informed about the latest developments in AI, particularly in healthcare, is crucial for healthcare professionals and the public alike.

This involves continuous learning, participation in workshops and conferences, and engagement with leading experts in the field.

The integration of AI into healthcare presents not just opportunities, but also challenges. As AI algorithms become more sophisticated, we must address the potential for bias, ensure patient privacy, and maintain human oversight of AI systems. Ethical considerations must be at the forefront of every development and application of AI in healthcare.

The future of healthcare is undeniably intertwined with AI. It's a future where AI empowers healthcare professionals, improves patient outcomes, and transforms healthcare systems. By embracing the potential of AI while navigating the challenges it presents, we can pave the way for a healthier future for everyone.

Imagine a world where AI-powered systems detect diseases in their earliest stages, allowing for timely interventions and preventing the development of serious complications.

Imagine personalized treatment plans tailored to individual needs, maximizing treatment effectiveness and minimizing side effects. Imagine a world where healthcare is more accessible, reaching underserved populations and bridging healthcare disparities. This is the potential that AI holds.

The journey toward this shared future requires a collective effort. By embracing collaboration, fostering innovation, and upholding ethical principles, we can harness the power of AI to transform healthcare and create a healthier world for everyone.

# Acknowledgments

This book would not have been possible without the invaluable contributions of many individuals. I am deeply grateful to the experts in Artificial Intelligence, Ethics, Psychology, and Sociology who collaborated with me on this project, sharing their knowledge, insights, and perspectives. Their guidance and expertise have shaped the book's content and deepened its understanding of the complex intersection of AI and human consciousness.

I am also indebted to my editor, [editor's name], for their meticulous attention to detail, insightful feedback, and unwavering support throughout the writing process. Their guidance has helped me to refine my ideas, clarify my arguments, and craft a more engaging and accessible narrative.

I would also like to thank the researchers, practitioners, and thought leaders who have generously shared their time, insights, and work with me. Their research and experiences have provided valuable context and inspiration for the book.

Finally, I am grateful to my family and friends for their unwavering encouragement and support, providing a much- needed source of inspiration and motivation during the long hours of writing.

# Afterword

The creation of "The N.E.R.D.Y. Way: An Everyday Guide to AI" was a collaborative effort, and we are deeply grateful to everyone who contributed their expertise, insights, and unwavering support.

First and foremost, we would like to express our sincere gratitude to the 3CAT team for their meticulous research, insightful contributions, and dedication to crafting engaging and accessible content. Their collective expertise and passion were instrumental in bringing this book to life.

We extend our heartfelt thanks to the reviewers who provided valuable feedback and guidance throughout the writing process. Their thoughtful suggestions and constructive criticism helped shape the book into its final form.

We are also grateful to the individuals and organizations who generously shared their knowledge and experience, contributing to the depth and accuracy of the book. Their insights have enriched the content and provided valuable context for our readers.

Finally, we would like to thank our families and friends for their patience and understanding during the long hours spent writing and editing this book. Their unwavering support has been a source of inspiration and strength.

This appendix provides additional resources and information to complement the content discussed in the book.

# APPENDIX & GLOSSARY

## APPENDIX

The appendix contains supplementary information that complements the main
content of the book.

### A.1: Glossary of AI Terms

This section provides definitions of key AI terms used throughout the book,
ensuring clarity and understanding for readers.

### A.2: Data Sources and Methodologies

This section details the data sources used to support the information presented
in the book, along with the
methodologies employed for analysis.

### A.3: Ethical Guidelines for AI in Healthcare

This section provides a summary of ethical guidelines and regulations related to
the use of AI in healthcare,
highlighting key considerations for responsible development and deployment.

### A.4: Resources for Further Exploration

This section lists valuable resources, including websites, articles, and organizations, that offer further information about AI in healthcare and related
fields.

# GLOSSARY

This glossary provides definitions for key terms and concepts discussed in the book, making it easier for readers to navigate the complex world of AI.

1. **Artificial Intelligence (AI):** The ability of a computer or machine to perform tasks that typically require human intelligence, such as learning, problem-solving, and decision-making.
2. **Machine Learning (ML):** A type of AI that enables computers to learn from data without explicit programming. ML algorithms identify patterns and make predictions based on data input.
3. **Deep Learning (DL):** A subset of ML that uses artificial neural networks with multiple layers to learn from complex data, such as images, text, and audio.
4. **Neural Network:** A computational model inspired by the structure and function of the human brain, consisting of interconnected nodes (neurons) that process and transmit information.
5. **Big Data:** Extremely large datasets that are often complex and unstructured, requiring advanced analytical tools to extract meaningful insights.
6. **Algorithm:** A set of instructions or rules used to solve a problem or perform a specific task.
7. **Data Mining:** The process of extracting valuable information from large datasets by using statistical and analytical techniques.
8. **Natural Language Processing (NLP):** A field of AI that focuses on enabling computers to understand and process human language.
9. **Computer Vision:** A field of AI that enables computers to "see" and interpret images and videos, similar to human vision.
10. **Robotics:** The field of engineering that deals with the design, construction, operation, and application of robots.
11. **Telemedicine:** The use of technology to provide healthcare services remotely, such as video consultations and remote monitoring.
12. **Electronic Health Records (EHRs):** Digital versions of patient medical records that store and manage health information electronically.
13. **Wearable Devices:** Devices that are worn on the body and collect

data about health and activity, such as fitness trackers and smartwatches.

14. **Predictive Analytics:** The use of data and statistical models to predict future events or outcomes.
15. **Personalized Medicine:** A healthcare approach that tailors treatment plans to the individual needs and characteristics of each patient.

# References & Sources

This section provides a list of references and sources that were consulted in the writing of this book.


1. Adler-Milstein J, Aggarwal N, Ahmed M, Castner J, Evans BJ, Gonzalez AA, James CA, Lin S, Mandl KD, Matheny ME, Sendak MP, Shachar C, Williams A. Meeting the moment: Addressing barriers and facilitating clinical adoption of artificial intelligence in medical diagnosis. NAM Perspectives. 2022;2022:10.31478/202209c. [PMC free article] [PubMed]
2. Baumol WJ, Bowen WG. On the performing arts: The anatomy of their economic problems. The American Economic Review. 1965;55(1/2):495–502.
3. Beatty C, Malik T, Meheli S, Sinha C. Evaluating the therapeutic alliance with a free-text CBT conversational agent (Wysa): A mixed-methods study. Frontiers in Digital Health. 2022;4:847991. [PMC free article] [PubMed]
4. Center for Medical Interoperability. Home page. 2021. [May 18, 2023]. https://medicalinteroperability.org/
5. Darcy A, Daniels J, Salinger D, Wicks P, Robinson A. Evidence of human-level bonds established with a digital conversational agent: Cross-sectional, retrospective observational study. JMIR Formative Research. 2021;5(5):e27868. [PMC free article] [PubMed]
6. Dosovitsky G, Bunge EL. Bonding with bot: User feedback on a chatbot for social isolation. Frontiers in Digital Health. 2021;3:735053. [PMC free article] [PubMed]
7. Fred HL, Gonzalo JD. Reframing medical education. Texas Heart Institute Journal. 2018;45(3):123–125. [PMC free article] [PubMed]
8. Hendrix N, Veenstra DL, Cheng M, Anderson NC, Verguet S. Assessing the economic value of clinical artificial intelligence:

Challenges and opportunities. Value in Health. 2022;25(3):331–339. [PubMed]

9. IOM (Institute of Medicine). Crossing the quality chasm: A new health system for the 21st century. Washington, DC: The National Academies Press; 2001. [PubMed]

10. Klein E. The New York Times. Mar 12, 2023. [June 23, 2023]. This changes everything. https://www.nytimes.com/2023/03/12/opinion/chatbots-artificial-intelligence-future-weirdness.html .

11. Lehne M, Sass J, Essenwanger A, Schepers J, Thun S. Why digital medicine depends on interoperability. npj Digital Medicine. 2019;2:79. https://doi.org/10.1038/s41746-019-0158-1 . [PMC free article] [PubMed]

12. Lim SM, Shiau CWC, Cheng LJ, Lau Y. Chatbot-delivered psychotherapy for adults with depressive and anxiety symptoms: A systematic review and meta-regression. Behavior Therapy. 2022;53(2):334–347. [PubMed]

13. Lomis K, Jeffries P, Palatta A, Sage M, Sheikh J, Sheperis C, Whelan A. NAM Perspectives. Washington, DC: National Academy of Medicine; 2021. [June 24, 2023]. Artificial intelligence for health professions educators. Discussion paper. https://nam.edu/artificial-intelligence-for-health-professions-educators/ [PMC free article] [PubMed]

14. Mantri Y, Jokerst JV. Impact of skin tone on photoacoustic oximetry and tools to minimize bias. Biomedical Optics Express. 2022;13(2):875–887. [PMC free article] [PubMed]

15. Matheny M, Thadaney Israni S, Ahmed M, Whicher D. Artificial intelligence in health care: The hope, the hype, the promise, the peril. Washington, DC: National Academy of Medicine; 2019. National Academy of Medicine special publication.

16. Mullainathan S, Obermeyer Z. Diagnosing physician error: A machine learning approach to low-value health care. Quarterly Journal of Economics. 2022;137(2):679–727.

17. National Academies of Sciences, Engineering, and Medicine; Health and Medicine Division; Board on Global Health; Global Forum on Innovation in Health Professional Education; Forstag EH, Cuff PA, editors. Artificial Intelligence in Health Professions Education:

Proceedings of a Workshop. Washington (DC): National Academies Press (US); 2023 Aug 14. References. Available from: https://www.ncbi.nlm.nih.gov/books/NBK598955/

18. Novak LL, Russell RG, Garvey K, Patel M, Thomas Craig KJ, Snowdon J, Miller B. Clinical use of artificial intelligence requires AI-capable organizations. JAMIA Open. 2023;6(2):ooad028. [PMC free article] [PubMed]

19. Obermeyer Z, Powers B, Vogeli C, Mullainathan S. Dissecting racial bias in an algorithm used to manage the health of populations. Science. 2019;366:447–453. [PubMed]

20. ONC and HHS (Office of the National Coordinator for Health Information Technology and the Department of Health and Human Services). 21st Century Cures Act: Interoperability, information blocking, and the ONC Health IT Certification Program. 2020. [June 23, 2023]. https://www.federalregister.gov/d/2020-07419/p-42de .

21. Russell RG, Lovett Novak L, Patel M, Garvey KV, Craig KJT, Jackson GP, Moore D, Miller BM. Competencies for the use of artificial intelligence-based tools by health care professionals. Academic Medicine. 2023;98(3):348–356. [PubMed]

22. Sendak MP, Gao M, Brajer N, Balu S. Presenting machine learning model information to clinical end users with model facts labels. npj Digital Medicine. 2020;3(1):41. [PMC free article] [PubMed]

23. Tyson A, Pasquini G, Spencer A, Funk C. 60% of Americans would be uncomfortable with provider relying on AI in their own health care. Pew Research Center; 2023. [June 23, 2023]. https://www.pewresearch.org/science/2023/02/22/60-of-americans-would-be-uncomfortable-with-provider-relying-on-ai-in-their-own-health-care/

24. Wachter R. The digital doctor: Hope, hype, and harm at the dawn of medicine's computer age. New York: McGraw-Hill Education; 2017.

25. Wu E, Wu K, Daneshjou R, Ouyang D, Ho DE, Zou J. How medical AI devices are evaluated: Limitations and recommendations from an analysis of FDA approvals. Nature Medicine. 2021;27(4):582–584. [PubMed]

# About the Author
## Dr. C.B. Howard, 3CAT

3CAT is a collective of professionals collaborating across various disciplines to offer innovative and practical solutions for individuals seeking to comprehend the effects of artificial intelligence (AI). We are committed to the dissemination of education and information, striving to enhance the lives of others. While knowledge is a powerful tool, its true potential is realized through its application.

At 3CAT, we acknowledge that everyone is unique. Consequently, we provide a diverse range of training and guidance materials tailored to accommodate different needs and learning preferences. Our publications cover a wide range of important topics, aiming to deepen understanding and knowledge in various areas of interest.

For every publication, 3CAT collaborates to conduct research, develop pertinent topics, create manuscripts, and oversee the publication process, to ensure the highest quality work possible.

The **N.E.R.D.Y.** WAY is an acronym for k**N**owledge, **E**ducation, **R**esource, **D**iscovery for **Y**ou.

*The trademark for "The NERDY WAY" has been applied for and is currently pending.*